LIVING OUT OF THE BOX

CHANGING THE FACE OF HEALTHCARE

Dr. Deborah Z. Bain, MD

Published in the United States by Platypus Publishing

Cover Design: Shahram Ayoubzadeh

Library of Congress Cataloging-in Publication Data:

ISBN# 978-1-962133-96-8

Author: Deborah Z. Bain, MD

Title: Living Out of the Box, Changing the Face of Heathcare

Description: 1st Edition, paperback

Subjects: Children's health, Advocacy

Table of Contents

Dedication

This book is dedicated to all those who are struggling with health problems and find themselves stuck in a medical system that seeks to manage their symptoms and not cure them.

My prayers go out to you for strength and courage for your journey.

It is my sincere hope that you will read something in these pages to inspire you to take the steps needed to improve your health.

Health is not just the absence of disease. It is living the kind of lifestyle that promotes and embraces it.

Carpe Diem!

Deborah Z. Bain, MD

Foreword

In my almost three decades of practicing medicine, I have become disheartened by the increasingly compartmentalized and fragmented healthcare system that I serve. Healthcare should mean more than just "disease-management care." The United States spends more dollars on healthcare than most nations do, and yet we are one of the sickest countries in the world. Children, for example, are now predicted to have a shorter life expectancy than their parents. Kids are being diagnosed with allergies, asthma, autism, ADHD, autoimmune disease, mental illness, cancer, obesity, and diabetes at alarmingly high rates. The most current surveillance statistics show that approximately 1 in 6 American children have been diagnosed with ADHD, 1 in 10 have anxiety, and 1 in 36 have autism, increased from 1 in 10,000 in the 1970's. Nearly 1 in 5 children (18.9%) have a seasonal allergy, 10.8% have eczema, 5.8% have a food allergy, and 6.5% have asthma (National Center for Environmental Health, 2023; Zablotsky et al., 2023). If you do the math, given the 2024 US population statistics showing 78 million children in the US, then just in America, ADHD affects 13 million children, anxiety 7.8 million, and autism 2.2 million, just to name a few. It does not have to be this way, but unfortunately, the current way of managing illness does not lend itself to the cure and reversal of these diseases. As I read pediatric medical journals and news brief publications, I cannot help but conclude that the focus of these articles is not to cure these kids of their chronic diseases, but rather to keep them "well managed." In America, we have quite the list of medications that can do just that, from antidepressants, stimulants, acid blockers, bronchodilators, antihistamines, to vaccinations to prevent just about anything from diarrhea to whooping cough. In my previous pediatric practice, it was not unusual for me to see a patient with a laundry list of medications that they were "well-managed on," just to have their annual checkup visit and request refills on their medications and referrals back to their specialists. But as I have learned throughout the years of practicing medicine, health is not just the absence of disease, nor does "well-managed" mean "well." I find it interesting that some parents have not even entertained the thought of being able to take their child off medication, and feel it is just normal to refill their child's drugs for, forever. They have been told that their child must have just inherited their parents' allergies and asthma, or tendencies for ADHD or autoimmune disease, and that is just the way it is. But the norm in my current integrative practice is that families are frustrated with their situation, their child's chronic need for medication and specialist referrals, and they are asking the tough questions: "Is this all I can expect for my child's health?

Is there another way? Can I ever get my child off these medications?" If you are one of these parents, then this book is for you, read on and be enlightened. If you are one of those skeptical, but curious parents or healthcare providers, I encourage you to open your mind and do not be quick to disregard the truths that will be revealed, not solely by evidence-based, double-blind placebo-controlled studies, but by well-intentioned, common-sense medicine based on my extensive training and experience in integrative and functional medicine. The stories in this book are real (although the names were changed to protect their privacy) and so are the struggles and frustrations these families have faced. These children did not get better with a one-size-fits-all approach to their symptoms. They were able to be freed from their reliance on medication by getting to the root cause of their illness. By applying a "thinking out of the box" approach, I was able to help even the most chronic, seemingly helpless disease state and make great strides in improving their health. By using a team of alternative and traditional practitioners, I was able to turn these kids' health around for the better.

I left the conformist approach to medicine nineteen years ago after going through my own health battles including nine neck and back surgeries in my early 30's and breast cancer at age 39. I tell my story in "How the Chiropractor Saved My Life, My Journey to Wellness and Beyond." I give thanks to my medical journey, for I would not be where I am today without it, nor would I have such great insight into helping others, as I do now.

****

I may not be where I intended to be,
but I know I ended up where I was meant to go.
Anonymous

"Living Out of the Box, Changing the Face of Healthcare" is a book of hope and advocacy for families searching for real health solutions, not just disease management. So read on and join me in "Living Out of the Box."

1

Defining the Box

"A problem cannot be solved on the level at which it appears. It must be solved on a higher level."

Albert Einstein

Consider with me the famous nine dots puzzle. The goal of the puzzle was to link all nine dots using four straight lines or less, without lifting the pen. The solution to the puzzle appears impossible only when you imagine a sort of artificial boundary around the edge of the dots themselves.

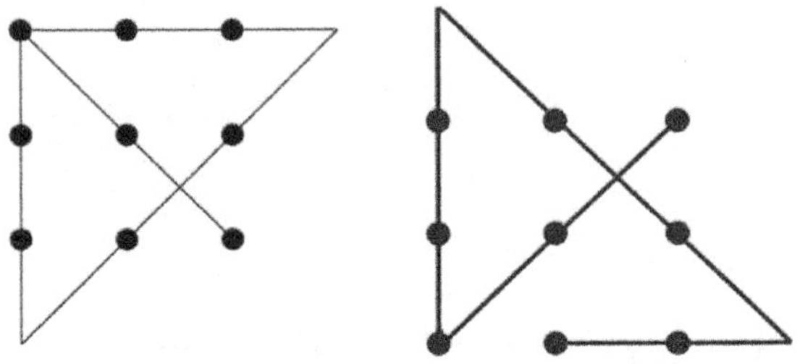

Image adapted from dottodotnametracing.com

Thinking “outside the box” then has been used as a metaphor for thinking differently, unconventionally, outside the boundaries, or from a new perspective. Thinking “inside the box" then, implies thinking that is conventional, traditional, and/or restrictive in nature.

Now I want you to imagine a more expanded definition of being in the box as it relates to healthcare. It can be considered oppressive, confining, restrictive and stiff to some, but may be considered safe, secure, and predictable to others. On another level, being in the box may represent the barriers in our lives that we create, walls we have constructed, defining ourselves or our children by their diagnosis that then perpetuates a way of thinking. “I am diabetic,” or “I am ADHD,” or “I am asthmatic.” These are just a few of the labels people present to my office with. In reference to the healthcare industry itself, this box has become an ominous structure with rigid unyielding walls, full of “standard-of-care protocols, management algorithms, procedures, and lots of red tape.

Let’s examine some of the personal "boxes" we might find ourselves in. Which one resonates with you the most?

One group of patients I see are those who are "content to stay in the box." They find the box symbolizing their current health management comfortable, predictable, and secure. The boundaries of this box don't feel too confined or restrictive to them. These patients are satisfied with managing their illness and symptoms, routinely refilling their prescriptions, and attending specialist follow-up visits. They comply with their doctor's advice and accept their guidance without hesitation, for who are they to question a medical authority? Whether or not their chronic condition is perfectly managed, as long as the disease doesn't significantly disrupt their livelihood, their symptoms are controlled with medication, they view their box as comfortable or at least tolerable.

Some of the content “in the box” patients may in truth be so numbed by the medical system that they do not even know how they got there. They wake up one day and realize they are on five different medications, seeing multiple specialists, all managing some set of symptoms, and all they wanted was to feel better. Since the medications work to some extent, they continue them, never getting any closer to the root cause of their seemingly unrelated ailments. The patients may not know the right questions to ask or what details are important to disclose to the doctor, and often are not given enough time to delve into their medical condition to really get back on track. So, the patient remains in a medically managed, sick state, and potentially forfeits any chance of becoming truly well.

This is much different than the second group of patients and families I see, who have been harmed in some way by the conventional medical system's approach to their care. To them, the box would be described as rigid, closed-minded, oppressive, lonely and dark. These are patients with chronically debilitating illnesses that are profoundly affecting their lives. These patients might suffer from chronic pain, cancer, autoimmune disease, severe eczema, allergies, recurrent ear infections, or autism, and they are frustrated by how their health has deteriorated despite following standard medical advice and attending all scheduled appointments intended to keep them well. These patients are determined to escape this box. They ask difficult questions, but the current medical system often fails to provide the answers they need. Their concerns are frequently dismissed or trivialized by conventional medical professionals. They may come to my office feeling either bitter and skeptical after hearing all the standard responses, or desperate and disheartened, clinging to a sliver of hope that their child can recover. They may have encountered doctors who, despite their impressive training from top medical schools and renowned professors, have become rigid in their approach, adhering strictly to protocols and pharmaceutical and surgical solutions, rather than exploring the root cause of the patient's disease state. Often these initial encounters end in a purging cry by a mother who falls into my arms as she finds hope for the first time. The medical paradigm that doctors have been taught, me included, is compartmentalized and fragmented in its approach. Medical schools continue to teach aspiring young doctors that a specific set of symptoms leads to a treatment plan that encompasses medications, procedures, and referrals to specialists. However, within these treatment protocols, there is often little to no emphasis on a comprehensive holistic approach that incorporates dietary changes, lifestyle modifications, and vitamin supplementation.

Research that drives medical decision-making for drug treatments of chronic illnesses often ignores underlying root cause contributors such as inflammatory diets and dysbiosis, and just focuses on the management of the disease. This leads to frustration among parents, who feel trapped in this oppressive box called the "healthcare system," and struggle to find a way out, to get "well," not to settle for being "well managed."

That is how I felt as a patient in the standard medical system as I went through 5 neck fusions and 4 lower back surgeries and then battled breast cancer, all in my 30s. I was faced with a one-sided way of treating my back and neck pain and weakness and that was medication, invasive procedures such steroid injections and burning of the nerve roots, and ultimately spinal fusion surgeries. I was made to feel fear, based on grim survival statistics, as a driving force to comply with chemotherapy and radiation treatments for my stage 3B breast cancer. I felt trapped and knew no other way back then, so I allowed these medical doctors to dictate these interventions on behalf of the best interest for my "health" or more accurately, to "stabilize my disease state." As I look back in retrospect, it was the system and its rigid treatment protocols that prevented any of my doctors from truly seeing my medical complaints in a holistic way. Not once did my orthopedic surgeon even question why my neck kept herniating above or below the fusion sites. To him it just happens, just the nature of the joint. Surely it couldn't be linked to my nutritional deficiencies or stress, or could it?

Breast cancer treatment was even more protocol driven, leaving me at the doctor's mercy as he reviewed the latest chemotherapy drugs and radiation treatments for my cancer. It was not until I broke out of this medical paradigm of a compartmentalized way of thinking that I could embrace ideals that led to my full recovery and state of wellness.

The third group of patients and families that I encounter are those who have successfully gotten out of the box. To these families, the box is also seen as rigid, confining, dark and oppressive but now it lays wide open, exposed, holes punched through letting light shine into it. To these people, they want to spread the message to the world on the way to get out of the box, to break free, to experience freedom and healing, to see the light. They want to break down those walls, tear off the red tape and rip that box wide open for others to see and for others to be freed. Once you "see" you cannot "unsee." It takes an open-minded person and an out of the box thinker to break down these barriers. As you can see, the only way you can solve that 9-dot puzzle is to have the lines reach outside the box constraints. That is the only way I can perceive that we are going to take charge of our health and really live a full life of wellness and not just be "well managed." We must stop considering the disease state as an end to itself, treated with a set of predictable medications and procedures. Instead, we need to see things as out of balance and look for ways to get back in balance before the disease state can occur. In doing so, a person does not live in fear of the inevitable disease just because they have a family history or genetic predisposition for it.

Let's face it, the medical industry itself is a business, and within that business comes smaller businesses such as hospitals, pharmaceutical supply companies, pharmacies, surgery centers, rehabilitation centers, speech and occupational therapy centers, etc. The healthcare industry by default lends itself to a sick model of medicine. If everyone is living a healthy lifestyle including eating healthy foods and exercising regularly, why would they need medication or surgery? These things should be considered the last resort when all other natural interventions have been exhausted, not first line – pop a pill for every ill and continue to live the lifestyle that got you into this mess in the first place. But sadly, that is the societal norm.

Integrative medicine doctors, me included, embrace a wellness model of medicine, encouraging people to take charge of their own health, to question their doctors about the side effects of medications and to ask about natural alternatives instead. However, we are the very doctors that are being called "quacks," cancelled, threatened and ridiculed by the medical community for our efforts to cure disease and not just manage it as the standard of care paradigm would dictate. But how can helping people reach a state of health and well-being and embracing wellness instead of furthering a disease state or prescribing nutritional supplements instead of medications be so wrong? Shouldn't our jobs as physicians be to give the patient the best chance to fully heal? We took an oath "primum non nocere" in Latin means first do no harm, however, I feel the doctors in this generation have been indoctrinated into the "system" they serve, and it is harder to have the autonomy to truly care for the patient as an individual, especially in the corporate or hospital-based practices who embrace protocol-driven medicine approaches. I believe integrative medicine doctors are forward-thinking pioneers and healers, not just practitioners.

Ignaz Semmelweis, a Hungarian physician and scientist of German descent in 1840's was a pioneer in antiseptic policy, considered a "savior of mothers" (Kadar et al., 2018). He introduced the concept of hand washing with a chlorinated lime solution before delivering babies. He showed decreased death rates from a common bacterial infection of the reproductive tract following birth called puerperal fever or childbed fever that was common and fatal. He was rejected by the medical community for his ideas. He became outspoken for his ideas about handwashing, but he could not produce a theoretical explanation for his findings. He suffered a nervous breakdown and was imprisoned in an insane asylum by his colleagues! In the asylum he was beaten by the guards and died two weeks later due to a gangrenous wound to his hand thought to have been caused by the beatings. Years later, Louis Pasteur proposed the germ theory which gave a theoretical basis and credibility to Dr. Semmelweis' observations. The evolution of medicine starts with a "rebel idea," that causes the creator to be ostracized for such a radical point of view, leading to an eventual reframing of the creator as a pioneer in their field, and then the idea becoming "standard of care."

Years ago, during a 3 month leave of absence for breast cancer treatment, I became determined to get well. The knowledge that I gained during that absence was eye-opening. I tried to implement some of my new-found knowledge in my previous corporate-owned practice, but it was not received well. I was told "you can't teach that here" and "you are different now and don't really fit our medical model anymore." I knew that the only way I could come back from my leave of absence and truly help people become well, was to open a holistic integrative pediatric practice to freely teach these principles of health and wellness. I left the corporate compliance rigid protocol-driven model of patient care and have never looked back. For someone who is inside the box, whether it be the patient or healthcare provider, or the medical system itself, or the medical institutions that support it, it is difficult to change that mindset because they are inside that dark box.

Here are some comments my patients submitted to me regarding their treatment by their prior healthcare provider when they did not want to follow the standard vaccine schedule for their child.

"I was talked down to as though I was ignorant, essentially told that people who modify schedules/don't vaccinate are responsible for all the disease in the world, and repeatedly pressured to change my decision, as well as guilted me like I was a bad mom for my decisions."

"I was bullied by my pediatrician and nurses, saying my child would suffer and get sick if I didn't give him shots.

"When I said I wanted to delay the schedule I was told – why inconvenience myself."

"When I moved to Texas the pediatrician was surprised that my son was so healthy and survived this long without all his shots."

"Every visit I was pestered, are we getting shots today? I felt bullied and harassed."

"I felt threatened."

"I was asked to leave the practice."

"I was ridiculed for wanting to modify my son's vaccination schedule."

"I have been demeaned, told not to come back, and made to feel like an idiot."

"One doctor threatened to turn me and my husband in for child neglect for refusing shots."

"I was fired from my pediatric practice for not complying with the standard vaccination schedule."

Can you relate to any of these patient quotes?

It is not right to alienate, shame, ridicule, or fire patients for not complying with an ever-changing vaccine schedule. I have many families that transferred care to my office due to a desire to have choice in medical decision making and true informed consent that was literally nonexistent in their current practice. I have heard many stories of moms being coerced in the operating room after a C-section birth to sign a form accepting the Hepatitis B vaccine to be given in the first 30 minutes of life for her baby, while being under the influence of anesthesia and pain medications, for the sake of the staff "not forgetting" to get it done. I take care of many other families who were told that "it is time for the 2-, 4- or 6-month shots" and the parent was not informed of what exactly their child was even receiving and were not given any freedom to deviate from the standard vaccination schedule. Instead, these families were fired from the pediatric practice for not complying with all the shots regardless of their state of health at the time they were due. They are horrified when they look at the vaccination printout of all the vaccines their child received. Parents feel trapped in the rigid box called our medical system and are fighting for their rights for choice in all healthcare decisions.

Over the last 29+ years of practicing medicine, I have seen hostility grow on this issue and many others regarding the care and treatment of children. How can we so easily ignore the growing population of chronically ill, nutritionally depleted children in our midst? How can we compartmentalize the administration of any medication or vaccination, injected or oral and say it does not affect a vulnerable immune system adversely? The question we should be asking is, “how can we ignore science?”

Parents are begging for a conversation about vaccines with their primary care provider to make an informed decision regarding protection of their child from vaccine preventable diseases, but instead are fed party-line, standard of care protocols and told to leave the practice if they do not comply. The vaccine schedule is daunting and confusing especially for new parents. Rather than feeling empowered to ask questions about vaccines, many parents, feeling stressed or uninformed, and by default, often choose to blindly trust their healthcare providers to accept all the "standard" vaccines. This can happen without realizing they have options to slow down or decline vaccines that don’t align with their lifestyle or risk levels. Conversely, some parents may feel paralyzed by uncertainty due to a lack of knowledge, leading them to take no action at all. Others, after conducting their own research, decide against vaccination entirely and are often labeled as "anti-vaxxers" in a derogatory manner by the medical community. The bottom line here is that having true informed consent and respecting body autonomy should be the standard approach to vaccine administration, not being pressured or coerced into compliance with an ever-growing vaccine schedule.

Hear what the CDC authorities say about vaccines and their contraindications vs. precautions regarding administration and ask yourself, does this make common sense? A contraindication to vaccination is a patient who has a condition that increases the risk for a serious adverse reaction to vaccination. (National Center for Immunization and Respiratory Diseases, 2023). Examples include severe allergic reactions or anaphylaxis to a vaccine or component of a vaccine and severe immunodeficiency. That's it. A precaution is a condition the person has that might increase the risk for a serious adverse reaction, cause diagnostic confusion if the vaccine is administered, or compromise the ability of the vaccine to produce an immune response. In this scenario, a person might experience a more severe reaction to the vaccine than would have otherwise been predicted. Examples here are people with autoimmune diseases, chronic illnesses, and acute or chronic infections. The CDC states that the "presence of a moderate to severe acute illness with or without fever is a precaution to administration of all vaccines," but that the patient should be vaccinated as soon as the acute illness has improved, including in hospitalized patients. The newest recommendations basically translate into vaccinating at every opportunity, during acute sick visits, hospital visits, well visits, and chronic care visits. To this point, I have often wondered why a hospitalized child with pneumonia is offered the flu vaccine and any other vaccines he is not up to date with, prior to discharge. Vaccine administration decisions should be based on current scientific evidence and personalized to the patient, not based on a protocol dictated by a pharmaceutical industry with limited liability for adverse reactions.

Neil Miller, founder of the Institute of Medical and Scientific Inquiry and founder and director of ThinkTwice Global Vaccine Institute has published multiple scientific papers and books on vaccine safety that deserve mention here. Although a controversial contributor to science by the mainstream who criticize Miller's lack of formal training, the papers he has published are solid in their content. Mr. Miller has observed through analysis of the VAERS data base a pattern regarding increased sudden infant deaths being temporally related to vaccine administration (Miller, 2021). Miller states that "although there is considerable evidence that a subset of infants has an increased risk of sudden death after receiving vaccines, health authorities eliminated *prophylactic vaccination* as an official cause of death, so medical examiners are compelled to misclassify and conceal vaccine-related fatalities under alternate cause-of-death classification." He goes on to say, "a review of the medical literature substantiates a link between vaccines and sudden unexplained infant deaths." Some of the proposed theories regarding the mechanism for which SIDS occurs after vaccine administration include, according to Miller's exhaustive research are "the role of inflammatory cytokines as neuromodulators in the infant medulla preceding an abnormal response to the accumulation of carbon dioxide; fatal disorganization of respiratory control induced by the adjuvants that cross the blood brain barrier; and biochemical or synergistic toxicity due to multiple vaccines administered concurrently." Miller's conclusion was that "while the findings in this paper are not proof of an association between infant vaccines and infant deaths, they are highly suggestive of a causal relationship." In a related article, Miller showed higher occurrences of severe allergies, autism, GI disorders, asthma, attention deficit disorders, and chronic ear infections in fully vaccinated and partially vaccinated as compared to unvaccinated (Hooker & Miller, 2020). The study also concluded the lowest incidence of adverse diagnoses in unvaccinated, breastfed infants as compared to highest incidence in fully vaccinated, not breastfed infants. Similarly lowest incidence of chronic diagnoses was found in vaginal births, unvaccinated versus cesarean section birth and fully vaccinated. Miller further makes the case that administering combinations of childhood vaccines at one visit is not safe (Miller, 2016). He showed that infants who receive "several vaccines concurrently...are significantly more likely to be hospitalized or die when compared with infants who receive fewer vaccines simultaneously." Assessment of the long-term effects of the current standard vaccination program on morbidity and mortality has been limited (Mawson, et al., 2016). In this controversial study comparing the health outcomes of vaccinated and unvaccinated homeschooled children, researchers observed lower odds of chickenpox and whooping cough among vaccinated children, as anticipated. However, they also found increased odds of conditions such as otitis media, pneumonia, allergies, and neurodevelopmental disorders (NDD), along with higher usage of medications, ear tube placements, and hospitalization in the vaccinated group. The suggested "dose-response" relationship between vaccination status and various chronic illnesses, along with the strong link between vaccination and NDDs, indicates that certain elements of the current vaccination program may be linked to increased risks of childhood morbidity. Notably, vaccination remained significantly associated with NDDs even after accounting for other variables, while preterm birth—previously viewed as a significant risk factor for NDD—showed no association when controlling for vaccination and other relevant factors. Additionally, the combination of preterm birth and vaccination appeared to significantly heighten the odds of NDD beyond the effects of vaccination alone.

Increased use of Acetaminophen appears to play a major role in the epidemic of autism, attention deficit disorder, and asthma in genetically vulnerable children (Shaw, 2013). Dr. Shaw addresses the scientific basis of a vulnerable detox pathway leading to an accumulation of a toxic metabolite called NAPQUI, causing reduced ability to detox from environmental chemicals, increased oxidative stress/free radical accumulation, and cellular and DNA damage. Dr. Shaw states in the article, "marked increases in the incidence of autism, asthma and attention deficit disorder in the United States coincide with the replacement of aspirin by acetaminophen in the 1980's. The characteristic loss of Purkinje cells in the brains of people with autism is consistent with depletion of brain glutathione due to excess acetaminophen usage, which leads to premature brain Purkinje cell death." With these novel facts in mind, I know from parents of children transferring care from other pediatric offices that their children were being pre-dosed with Acetaminophen prior to receiving vaccinations to prevent "post-vaccine fever," thereby avoiding that dreaded after-hours phone call, and thus unknowingly putting that patient at risk for adverse vaccine reactions!

To state the obvious, it is the person you are putting the medication or vaccination into that is the problem regarding adverse reactions. We need to ensure, to our best ability, that for any elective vaccination, the child's immune system is healthy to give them the best opportunity to respond normally to it. Although the concepts “overdosing” in the medical arena or concepts of “overdoing it” or “overindulging” make sense for other aspects in our lives, it is ignored or pragmatically denied in any vaccination discussion. A one-sized-fits-all model for vaccines frankly just does not make common sense. We calculate dosages for all other medications, why not vaccines. Family genetics, medical history, state of health, and nutritional status of the child should all be considered for every vaccine decision. At my holistic integrative pediatric practice, we educate families on alternatives to Acetaminophen including natural immune system support supplements such as homeopathic remedies to give the best chance for a healthy immune response to vaccinations, as well as give parents choice to accomplish a modified, selective, or delayed schedule.

The current medical paradigm or mindset is flawed. We are not sitting ducks waiting for a disease to take us out. A paradigm shift needs to occur that embraces a patient-centered wellness model of healthcare, and not a Band-aid fix approach to illness and disease. It will be up to everyone involved to open their mind, step out of the box, and work together to achieve a common goal – optimal health. The new norm should be allopathic doctors working with naturopaths, nutritionists, chiropractors, and other holistic practitioners to design complementary approaches for every condition, focusing on identifying imbalances in the body before a disease state occurs. If you wait for that heart attack to happen, you are going to need the best surgeons, nurses, and the best life-saving medications and medical interventions, but that should be a rare occurrence. Instead, we should be focusing on how to prevent heart attacks with programs that focus on nutrition, exercise, lifestyle, as well as supplementation for vitamin deficiencies, not just managing symptoms with blood pressure and cholesterol lowering medications.

2

Modern Day Canaries

"The level of civilization attained by any society will be determined by the attention it has paid to the welfare of its children."

B.F. Andrews

From the Children's Bill of Rights, 1968

Our children are the new modern-day canaries. Just like the canaries in the coal mines in the 1950's that alerted the coal miner the air was fit to breathe – or not, our children are giving us clear signals that they are in trouble and need our help!

Let me tell you about Nicholas. He is a now healthy, energetic 7-year-old but that is not how he presented to my office two years earlier. Nicholas had a long list of medical problems including recurrent ear infections, croup, colic and gastroesophageal reflux disease, all manifesting in the first year of life. He received his first set of vaccines on the standard schedule at 2 months of age including DTaP, Hib, Prevnar, IPV, Rotavirus and Hepatitis B. In the weeks that followed, he had almost constant spitting up, recurrent fevers, constant nasal congestion and fussiness. In the next several months he was plagued with recurrent ear infections requiring multiple courses of antibiotics. He had a second set of the same vaccinations at the age of 1 year, but almost immediately following, he developed loose stools/diarrhea as well as thrush and yeast skin infections, not surprising given the multiple courses of antibiotics he had received. No suggestions for help restoring gut flora were ever discussed by their pediatrician. Quite the contrary occurred for this family. When the parent asked the question about the use of probiotics, the pediatrician answered saying, "well you can spend your money if you want to, but it won't help." At 17 months of age, Nicholas had a third set of vaccines that included MMR, Varicella, Hepatitis A, and Hepatitis B, and approximately 45 minutes later, he started to scream, thrash around and bang his head against the floor and walls. Mom says the screams haunt her to this day. The screaming and writhing lasted four hours. The pediatrician's office told her it was just a tantrum, but mom knew it wasn't. She finally got him in the car which helped him to fall asleep, but it did not last, and he awoke and continued to scream for 3 more hours.

Nicholas also developed multiple sensory issues that became more obvious as he got older. He would come unglued when he had to switch from long sleeves to short sleeves or shorts when the season changed. He could not stand having his hair touched, combed or washed, and forget about being cut! Water on his face would send him into hysterics. He also had issues with textures. Unlike typical babies who love foods like bananas, yogurt, applesauce and oatmeal, he hated all things mushy in texture. He would only eat foods that were crunchy and formed. He practically lived off black beans, but they had to be whole, rinsed and plain.

Nicholas did not have any sense of fear or danger about his surroundings. Once he learned how to walk and run, he would follow his feet wherever they would take him. Going out in public became a safety threat because he would run off. At the age of 3 years, he still could not say or respond to his name, so if he was to get lost, he would not be able to ask for help. Parents resorted to placing a sticker on Nicholas' back with their cell phone numbers just in case. Nicholas could not handle the sensation of being suspended in the air, whether it was in a dentist's chair, on escalators, in glass elevators, on glass balconies in the mall, or walking up open staircases. Mom brought these concerns up to her pediatrician who just thought he would grow out of it. But mom finally knew something was seriously wrong when Nicholas started eating random non-food items. He started eating bars of soap, sticks of deodorant, shampoo, dirt, etc. Mom asked her pediatrician at the time if he could be tested for heavy metals. He said that the only heavy metals that he could test for were lead and iron. He was tested and found to have severe iron deficiency anemia, so he was placed on an iron supplement. He was also referred to a therapy center for a speech and occupational therapy evaluation for his sensory issues and was diagnosed with Pervasive Developmental Disorder with suspicion of Autism. Mom knew that there was more to his pica (eating of non-food items) and sensory issues than just iron deficiency.

Mom went in search of answers, and she found my holistic integrative pediatric practice. She finally found ears that would listen and tests that could somehow explain his laundry list of health concerns.

I introduced to her a concept that was so foreign to mom but at the same time made so much sense. First I reviewed his full history, obtained a detailed review of symptoms with the use of a medical symptom questionnaire, but then told his story back to mom with a functional medicine perspective.

Next I discussed terms such as dysbiosis, malabsorption, food sensitivities, possibly resulting in the evolution of nutrient depletion, increased total toxic burden contributing to evolution of many predictable medical problems including recurrent otitis (ear infections), rhinitis (allergies), dermatitis (eczema, keratosis pilaris), bronchitis (asthma), enteritis (Crohn's and Celiac Disease, Ulcerative Colitis), arthritis, vasculitis (POTS), thyroiditis (autoimmune Graves' disease and Hashimoto's disease), encephalitis (neurocognitive and neurobehavioral problems including motor tics, seizures, sensory processing disorder, pervasive developmental delays, autism, ADHD, anxiety and depression), and a weakened immune system in general.

I gave mom a handout which I created as a visual representation of my functional medicine training called the "Cycle of Illness" and the "7Rs of Healing Program." Just seeing this concept of the evolution of chronic disease on paper caused her to burst in tears saying, "why don't other doctors know this?" I also explained the 7Rs of Healing to systematically help reverse and improve symptoms and signs of any chronic disease state.

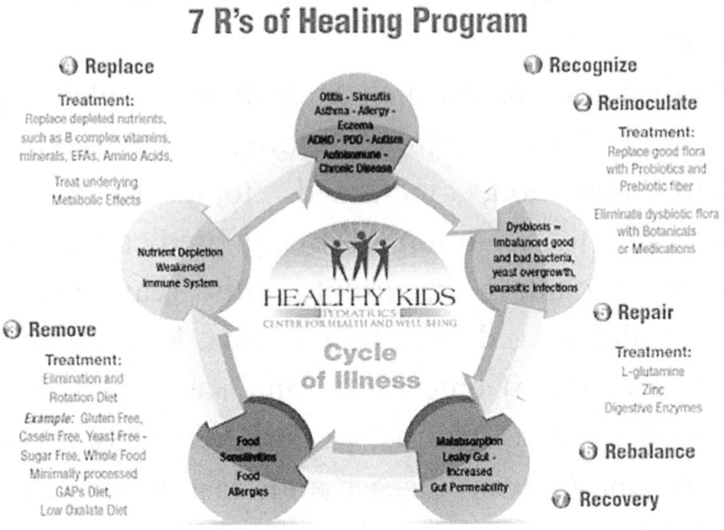
7 R's of Healing Program
Replace
Treatment:
Replace depleted nutrients, such as B complex vitamins, minerals, EFAs, Amino Acids,
Treat underlying Metabolic Effects
Recognize
Reinoculate
Treatment:
Replace good flora with Probiotics and Prebiotic fiber
Eliminate dysbiotic flora with Botanicals or Medications
Nutrient Depletion Weakened Immune System
Dysbiosis = Imbalanced good and bad bacteria, yeast overgrowth, parasitic infections
HEALTHY KIDS
CENTER FOR HEALTH AND WELL-BEING
Cycle of Illness
Remove
Treatment:
Elimination and Rotation Diet
Example: Gluten Free, Casein Free, Yeast Free - Sugar Free, Whole Food Minimally processed GAPs Diet, Low Oxalate Diet
Repair
Treatment:
L-glutamine
Zinc
Digestive Enzymes
Food Allergies
Leaky Gut - Increased Gut Permeability
Rebalance
Recovery

"Cycle of Illness & 7R's of Healing" Deborah Z. Bain, MD, 2016

It all starts with Recognize "-itises" are, for the most part, reversible, especially when discovered early. Next is to Re-inoculate with probiotics to reestablish healthy gut flora especially after c-section birth or courses of antibiotics. Third is Remove unhealthy foods and pathogenic yeast and bacteria, as well as parasites. Fourth is Replace healthy foods, macro and micronutrients. Fifth is Repair at the cellular and gut level. Sixth is Rebalance the immune system response and inflammation. Lastly is Recover to a healthier state of being. I warned mom that I may not be able to recover her child fully, but that I knew I could identify and address his unique imbalances, and then let his body do the rest. For the first time in mom's journey, she finally found hope.

I ordered a full nutritional analysis, comprehensive stool testing and IgE food allergy and IgG food sensitivity testing. He had severe B12, zinc, Magnesium, CoQ10, Vitamin C and Omega 3 essential fatty acid deficiencies. He had signs of yeast and bacterial dysbiosis, malabsorption, oxidative stress, low glutathione, elevated mercury, impaired methylation and mitochondrial dysfunction. His stool analysis showed signs of yeast as well as inadequate good bacterial flora and low secretory IgA – meaning his gut immune system was inadequate. He had no food allergies, but did have a few sensitivities to dairy, pecan and sesame. So basically, Nicholas had a huge toxic burden with his detox pathways essentially "offline" and malabsorption of the very nutrients he needed to reverse the oxidative stress on his body. I placed him on probiotics, high potency multivitamin, Omega 3 EFA, additional CoQ10, Vitamin C, Magnesium and zinc. He had a nutritionist consultation and ongoing follow-ups that were tailored just for him. Two years later at 6 years of age, he no longer qualified for speech or occupational therapy services! He transitioned well to kindergarten where he learned to read, write, do math, and make friends. Mom says he loves math, puzzles, mazes, building Legos and riding his bike without training wheels. He loves to retell stories with entertaining facial expressions and dramatic flair. He still has some quirky behaviors, and a bit of social immaturity compared to his peers, but what a journey back to wellness he has had.

Nicholas' story points out the fact that every child is unique in their genetics, gut flora, nutritional status, detoxification abilities, and overall capacity to handle what comes their way. When I see pictures of this adorable little red-headed child, smiling with his whole face, eyes piercing right through you, I cannot help but think what could have happened if mom did not start questioning "why?" Nicholas had such a picky palate and limited foods he would eat, not unlike so many other children I care for. So, logic will tell you that if we continue to overburden these kids with more medications, aggressive vaccination schedules, environmental pollutants, etc. that exceeds their ability to detox from, not to mention offering them highly processed foods devoid in macro and micronutrients, they can have similar symptoms as Nicholas.

I am a proponent of early nutritional and genetic testing on children, especially those with concerning family histories, to better determine treatment plans. If we can predict for example that a child has detoxification pathway abnormalities inherited from one or both parents, nutrient deficiencies, or mitochondrial dysfunction, then we can have an opportunity as a medical provider to choose to modify medical interventions and provide extra support during courses of medication, vaccination or surgical procedures involving anesthesia, to best protect the child from adverse reactions. It is well established that a family history of autoimmune disease or neuropsychiatric disorder increases the risk of similar abnormalities in children. If we know we have a trigger plus a genetic predisposition for certain disease states, then we have a potential perfect storm for a predictable adverse outcome. We are 99.9% genetically the same, and it is only 0.1% that varies between every person on this planet. So, if our genetics have not changed, and we are seeing an enormous increase in all chronic diseases, then one must conclude that our environment is playing a very large role in the development of these diseases.

A recent article in "The Defender" reported on a 62-day old infant who received the standard 2-month vaccines was found dead within 34 hours of the vaccine administration (Dumais, 2023). The interview of the parents pointed to their struggles to investigate the cause of death with being denied by the medical examiner to perform confirmatory lab toxicology testing to possibly point to a vaccine causation of this baby's death. The initial cause of death was reported as "asphyxiation due to inappropriate sleep position and environment." Parents knew this was not true and pursued a private toxicologist to investigate their child's death. Testing confirmed lethal amounts of aluminum as the cause of death for this baby. Baby Sawyer also reportedly had a viral rash that started one week prior to the vaccines and was present still at the time the vaccines were administered. Parents were hesitant to go through with the vaccines due to the rash but felt pressured to comply with the standard childhood immunization schedule and ultimately conceded to the injections due to the reassurance of the pediatrician.

In approximately 20 percent of VAERS (Vaccine Adverse Event Reporting System) reports, the top side effects listed suggest central nervous system involvement including "screaming, agitation, apnea, ataxia, visual disturbances, convulsions, tremors, twitches, an abnormal cry, hypotonia, hypertonia, abnormal sensations, stupor, somnolence, neck rigidity, paralysis, confusion, and oculogyric crisis (Orient, 1999)." Children, given their low body weights and their kidney function not fully developed until two years of age, are more likely to experience aluminum toxicity compared to their older peers (Lyons-Weiler et al., 2020). The author describes a "PDL - Pediatric Dose Limit" formula of aluminum in the study, showing graphs of exceeding limits based on age and the vaccine schedule followed. The conclusions of the paper suggest that "whole body aluminum toxicity from vaccines in infants from birth to six months indicate the CDC's recommended vaccination schedule leads to unacceptable long periods of time in which infants are in aluminum toxicity." Therefore, "careful consideration of expected aluminum exposures during regular and catch-up vaccination is found to be especially important for infants and children below 2 years of age." In a related article, a large observational study showed a positive association between vaccine related aluminum exposure and persistent asthma by way of skewing the immune system to a TH2 and away from a TH1 response (Daley et al., 2023).

Is it possible that the epidemic of neuro-developmental disorders, allergy, asthma, autoimmune disease, and sudden infant death syndrome could in part be due to the "standard" vaccine schedule which may exceed the maximum "safe" amount of aluminum, depending on how many vaccines were given at one time? How many other SIDS deaths may have been attributed to vaccination if only the question was raised or if raised did not fall on deaf ears. Factors such as low birth weight, genetic detox pathway mutations, low kidney function under 6 months of age, and pre-dosing of Acetaminophen prior to vaccination, should all be taken into consideration. A one-size-fits-all model just does not work. This is why an integrative, holistic medical approach is so important. Our focus should be on ensuring these children are nutritionally sound prior to electively vaccinating on the standard schedule. Standards are relative since they vary from state to state and from country to country. We should also be focusing on minimizing and eliminating toxins of all types including those *ingested* such as hydrogenated trans fats, artificial colors and sweeteners, *inhaled* such as airborne pollutants, topically *absorbed* through the skin in makeup, cleaning products, and soaps, and *injected.* We should be focusing on what we are putting into our bodies, encouraging a whole food, minimally processed, nutrient dense diet. Optimizing nutrition has been proven to improve any altered health state for the better, and most definitely poor nutrition and eating habits have contributed greatly to the epidemic of all chronic diseases in the world today.

Another tool I use in my office to illustrate this point is the "Liver Detox handout." It explains Phase I and Phase II detox and nutrient requirements needed at each step.

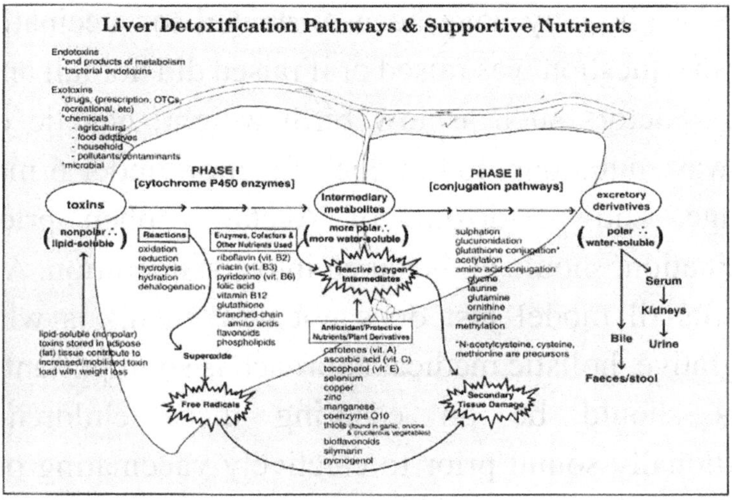

Image adapted from semanticscholar.org

In short, anything inhaled, injected, taken orally, or applied to or absorbed by the skin must potentially be detoxed from a fat-soluble into a water-soluble form to be excreted in the urine and stool (Phase III detox).

So many things can go wrong in this process from too much "toxin" coming in, to nutrient deficiencies at Phase I or II, or even constipation or dehydration and kidney function affecting Phase III detox. In my functional medicine training, we were often shown the classic "I Love Lucy chocolate factory episode" to provide a visual of this concept. In this episode, Lucy and Ethel must wrap chocolates coming down the conveyor belt. It was not too hard when the conveyor belt was slow and the number of chocolates on it was manageable. Obviously, it did not go well when the conveyor belt was purposely sped up and the number of chocolates on the conveyor belt increased! If you want a good laugh, you should watch the short YouTube video of this fiasco online. In much the same way, your body can be overburdened when forced to process too many toxins too quickly.

Jordan Rubin is one of America's most recognized and respected natural health experts, author of "The Maker's Diet," "Live Beyond Organic," and "Patient Heal Thyself," and founder of Garden of Life, a leading whole food nutritional supplement company. He is a proponent of non-GMO, organic foods and passionately writes about how dangerous genetically modified foods are to our bodies. GMO technology in the US has been used to make crops resistant to chemical herbicides such as Glyphosate, leading to an exponential increase in herbicide use (Abrams et al., 2024). Chemical companies have quite the monopoly on American and worldwide agriculture, selling

GM seeds and their GM-seed-taylored herbicides as packaged deals to farmers. These genetically modified seeds cannot regerminate, causing the farmer to be dependent upon a new supply of seeds every year. Genetically modified, tampered-with foods take genes from completely different species of plant or animal and splice them to DNA of the desired plant or animal. GM crops commonly encountered include corn, soy and dwarf wheat. Stephanie Seneff, PhD has been very outspoken regarding the disruptive effects of the herbicide, glyphosate on the body (Seneff, 2021).

1. Glyphosate is a very efficient metal chelator. That said, it may worsen the adverse effects of vaccines due to binding aluminum, an adjuvant used in many vaccines.
2. Glyphosate disrupts gut microbiome by binding to minerals which are needed by the microbes for enzyme production.
3. Glyphosate is a synthetic amino acid and is an analogue of glycine which is one of three amino acids that make glutathione, the body's #1 antioxidant needed for detoxification. Glyphosate binds to the glycine receptor, thus displacing glycine and in doing so is incorporated into peptides during protein synthesis, thus inhibiting the detoxification process.

In a related article, "glyphosate substitution for conserved glycines can easily explain a link with diabetes, adrenal insufficiency, hypothyroidism, Alzheimer's disease, amyotrophic lateral sclerosis, Parkinson's disease, prion diseases, lupus, mitochondrial disease, non-Hodgkin's lymphoma, neural tube defects, infertility, hypertension, glaucoma, osteoporosis, fatty liver disease, and kidney failure" (Samsel & Seneff, 2016).

I have seen first-hand based on the comprehensive nutrient testing I order in children with chronic diseases, very low levels of glycine and moderate to high need for glutathione amongst a plethora of other nutrient deficiencies. Not only do we have to worry about chemical and pharmaceutical companies controlling our entire food chain, but we also must worry about the pollutants in the air we breathe and the water we drink. We live in an incredibly toxic world. Even the clothing we wear, mattresses we sleep on and the carpets we walk on have been treated with multiple chemicals that can potentially threaten the health of a chemically sensitive, genetically vulnerable person.

The Environmental Working Group study on placental cord blood demonstrated nothing less than a toxic cesspool that the babies are bathing in prior to birth from all the petrochemicals, phthalates, cleaning products, etc. the mom had been exposed to in the environment (Houlihan et al., 2005). Clearly, since our genetics have remained unchanged, it must be our exposure to environmental toxins from various sources that is contributing to the rise in chronic diseases among both children and adults.

Brian is another one of those modern-day canaries. He started seeing me when he turned 3 years old. He had a diagnosis of developmental delay, sensory processing disorder, and dyspraxia. Mother said that he would have fever, fussiness and lethargy after his vaccinations and was told to give him Acetaminophen by their pediatrician. When he received his flu vaccine, he again developed fever and fussiness, but this time it was eerily different. He became physically sick, but even more distressing, he lost all verbal skills. How does a parent fathom such a thing? One minute your child is stringing phrases together and the next he is having incoherent babble. Could it be he received a toxic dose of aluminum from the multi-dose vial that was not properly shaken? At his 3-year checkup at my office he could not demonstrate any color or shape recognition, did not sing songs or count, could say only a few phrases, and was far from conversational. He was sensory seeking, loved to climb, stomp, and hit, spin in a swing with his head tilted, but could not tolerate physical touch especially of his head and could not pedal a tricycle due to being bothered by the spikey pedals. His past medical history was significant for being born at 38.5 weeks by emergency C-section after a failed induction which resulted in heart rate deceleration, poor color, and low Apgar scores at birth. He had jaundice and poor feeding initially, was only able to breast feed for two weeks, tried multiple formulas which he spit up, was diagnosed with formula intolerance, acid reflux that was treated with an acid-blocking medication. He was also eventually diagnosed with allergies and ear infections requiring pressure equalizing tubes at 17 months. Mom stopped vaccinating Brian after the 15-month shots because she knew something was not right. She began doing research on her own and started a multivitamin supplement at 24 months old, enrolled him in occupational and speech therapy at 25 months, and stopped dairy and gluten at 30 months. It was not until mom eliminated gluten that she saw Brian register a pain response to being hurt. Prior to that, she said he rarely cried and showed little or no discomfort with teething or ear infections.

Mom was desperate for answers and guidance when she had her first appointment. She was beyond frustrated at a system of healthcare that just served to medicate and manage her child's symptoms but provided no true guidance on getting her son well. It was an eye-opening moment for mom when I retold his story from a holistic perspective. I discussed the cycle of illness handout pointing out the pattern of gut dysbiosis, malabsorption, food sensitivities, contributing to nutritional deficiencies and evolution of neurocognitive and neurobehavioral problems, as well as eczema, asthma, allergies, and a weakened immune system in general. That was one power-packed statement for anyone to digest, but it made all the sense in the world! He nwas born by C-section, meaning he was brought into the world in a sterile environment, did not have the chance for gut colonization with a vaginal birth, breast fed only briefly after mom was also given intrapartum antibiotics. This scenario alone can lead to predictable formula intolerance to develop, especially when the formula chosen did not have probiotics and she was not informed that probiotics are essential for healthy gut flora. Seventy percent of the immune system is housed in the gut. There are more messages from gut to brain than brain to gut. So, if the gut immune system is compromised, so is the neurotransmitter production, detoxification system, absorption of nutrients, etc. After explaining this scenario, it was like an epiphany moment for mom. She welled up with tears and for the first time in her journey, she was filled with hope that she was on the right path to breaking free from the constraints of the oppressive "box" she had found herself in for the last three years. I stressed the importance of speech and occupational therapy as well as a biomedical approach to optimize Brian's developmental potential. I recommended comprehensive nutritional testing and food sensitivity and allergy testing. The results of the testing confirmed that he had moderate antioxidant and key vitamin/mineral deficiencies, severe Vitamin D deficiency, high yeast and bacterial dysbiosis, methylation and mitochondrial dysfunction, and essential fatty acid imbalances. He also had persistent markers for dairy intolerance even though he was eating a dairy-free diet. I placed him on Vitamin D3, a multi-strain probiotic 25 billion cfu chewable, an all-inclusive liquid multivitamin and mineral supplement, and an essential fatty acid omega 3 supplement. Nothing fancy was done, but the results of some simple attention to nutrition and detoxification support were profound.

Mom was beaming ear to ear at a follow-up appointment just 2 months later. She reported that the occupational therapists and other parents and teachers were asking her "what did you do to him…, what testing did you do…, what supplements is he taking?" He had made amazing progress in just two short months. He was so much more engaged and verbal. He was now able to sing songs, knew his alphabet and numbers, and was able to show imaginary play and interact normally with neuro-typical children. He found a love for music and sings to songs downloaded on mom's phone. Mom said that she was now able to completely cut his hair with distraction, something she would never have accomplished just a few months prior.

This is a testimony to paying attention to foundational nutrition, support of the body's needs for nutrients for running all the complex processes in the body including detoxification, minimizing exposures to toxicants, and the amazing ability of the body to reset and recover. It is so rewarding for me to guide these families through their unique journeys to help their little kids back to thriving, and to know that I have helped them break free from the grips of some state of disease or disorder, committed to therapies and medications with no end in sight. Where is the hope in that? Here we are one of the richest nations, and yet our healthcare system with its focus on disease care is making us sicker. This sick paradigm of compartmentalized medicine, even on this level, does not really pan out as an approach to a way of life that would embrace wellness and a cure or restoration to a normal state of being. The continuance of this sick medical paradigm benefits only the pharmaceutical companies, as they have much to lose if everyone is healthy and do not need their medications. I can say wholeheartedly that I can never go back to that dark, closed-minded, in the box approach to medicine.

My mother used to say, it is a good thing you could afford to get well from cancer. You know, I pondered about that a lot. For you see, there are so many people who are sick and cannot afford to get well. The current medical paradigm supports this sick model of medicine including management of disease with generic prescription medications, specialist visits, procedures and even surgery, all mostly paid for by insurance. It is easier for families to just fill a prescription at minimal cost than to do expensive nutrition testing. It is also easier for the family to buy cheap processed foods on sale than it is to buy organic foods and fresh produce for their family, thus perpetuating the problem, making them even more sick because the food itself is toxic to their bodies. This perpetual sick model of medicine is so far reaching, the next generation is guaranteed to be as sick, or sicker than the previous one, thus making more future customers for the medical industry. That is unless we collectively interrupt this paradigm. So as my mother said, yes, I could afford to get well; I could afford to go to the chiropractor, to purchase multiple supplements that my body was so deficient in after all my surgeries and breast cancer. It is sad to say, but my cancer and back and neck surgeries cost me nothing but copays, having minimal impact on our family budget, but it cost the medical system over 1.5 million dollars. It has cost me much more financially to get well, but you cannot put a price on health. Sure, it was much less expensive to take a prescription pill, but I cannot even begin to tell you the ultimate toll these interventions took on my health, physically and emotionally, as well as on my family through the struggles. I would have preferred healthier options to prevent my disease state than to have to go through such horrendous pain and suffering.

Investing in your health is the best thing you can do for yourself and for the generations to come. You and your family are worth it. It is worth it to buy that fresh or frozen organic produce instead of pesticide-laden produce. It is worth buying hormone free, non-genetically modified animal products. It is worth cooking hot healthy meals at home instead of relying on restaurants or fast foods cooked in hydrogenated fats. You see, the TV dinners or highly refined foods you buy do taste good, and do put food on the table, but at a price. Your job as a parent is to teach the next generation how to be well, making a habit of family meals and balanced nutrition. But when no one taught you how to be well, and your parents before them did not do the same, you can see how this cycle of illness has been perpetuated. Instead, parents are relying on the food industry itself to teach them what is healthy. Do you really trust commercials or advertisements to tell you what is healthy? I laugh when I see the old TV commercials on breakfast cereals as it states that the sugary cereal is "part of a nutritious breakfast" as they show the cereal surrounded by a glass of juice, piece of fruit, egg, and whole grain toast. Obviously, an advertising trick or market ploy to get you to buy their product, not telling you that the cereal was really the least healthy part, and debatable on everything else shown except maybe the piece of fruit and egg!

It is so troubling how, once the medical community finds out you are an Integrative doctor, they often assume you no longer follow traditional practices that they can relate to. Instead of belonging to the "good-old-boys club" feeding them much needed referrals, you are perceived as a lifestyle-focused, quasi-medicine practitioner. But in my opinion, I am and will always be a board-certified pediatrician first, and integrative medicine board certified doctor second. I did not throw out all the knowledge I acquired, but instead I brought more insight, experience, and perspective to the table than I did in the years of practicing so-called traditional medicine. I never stop learning ways to help my patients. It has never been so obvious to me that all our disciplines need to work together to raise a healthier next generation. We do not need to focus on our differences, but rather come to some common ground to move the practice of medicine forward into the 21st century.

3

A New Paradigm

"When health is absent, wisdom cannot reveal itself, strength cannot fight, intelligence cannot be applied, art cannot become manifest, wealth becomes useless."

Greek Physician Herophilus

"The part can never be well unless

the whole is well."

Plato

One of the most compelling, current problems in medicine is the failure of the conventional model medical diagnosis and treatment to successfully address the burden of chronic disease. The current allopathic medical system is not set up to adequately address the needs of chronically ill children, leaving them without sufficient solutions or support. Another observation that I have made is that if a child does not align with a specific checklist of symptoms and confirmatory exam results, diagnosing and determining the appropriate treatment can become a diagnostic dilemma. Take for instance a child with Juvenile Idiopathic Arthritis that I had the privilege of treating in an out-of-the-box way. The definition of "idiopathic" is "having no known cause," which tells a lot regarding how this case was handled by the "in-the-box" specialists.

Ashley was 8 years of age when she came to me with a history of trouble making a fist that then progressed to the inability to open a bag of chips or a peanut butter jar. When I first saw Ashley, she said her joints had become so painful and frozen that she had to literally crawl into the bathtub just to take a bath. Another clue to her diagnosis was her extensive family history of autoimmune disease and her atrocious diet containing only processed carbs, dairy, and gluten containing grains. On examination, she had a large, depigmented patch on her abdomen and leg consistent with vitiligo. She had very poor dentition with many cavities and extensive keratosis pilaris, otherwise known as "KP" or "chicken skin" on her face, arms, and legs. She had very stiff joints in her hands, wrists, elbows, knees, and ankles.

I referred her to a Rheumatologist for further evaluation but told her parents to put Ashley on a gluten-free, dairy-free diet while I ordered labs. KP is often associated with gluten and dairy sensitivity, the very foods she ate daily, as well as Omega 3 essential fatty acid deficiencies, contained in foods of which she never ate. The specialist evaluation concluded that she had JIA (Juvenile Idiopathic Arthritis) and said that it was an immune mediated condition, and the only treatment was medication to "halt inflammation." In their correspondence to me was an interesting notation stating that Ashley's symptoms had reportedly improved since she had been started on a gluten and dairy-free diet prescribed by her pediatrician. This fact was later ignored and treated as a curious coincidence. Instead of monitoring for more improvements following a natural approach, she was given a dose of Methotrexate on the spot, and her parents were told that the side effects may include liver toxicity, hair loss, nausea, abdominal pain and the potential for developing cancer!

The specialty labs done through my office concluded that Ashley had negative rheumatoid factor antibodies, significant B complex deficiencies, zinc deficiency, essential fatty acid imbalances, very low nutritionally essential amino acids and detoxification impairments, as well as high gluten and dairy sensitivities. The treatment plan was simple - gluten-free, dairy-free diet, optimize micro and macro nutrients as well as omega 3 essential fatty acids through supplementation and diet. In just a few months her joint stiffness had improved greatly, and she was beaming with joy as she could now do those little things that were almost impossible for her to do before. Was it the one magical Methotrexate dose that turned her condition around? I think not. Chronic illnesses require a comprehensive look at all factors including family history, diet history and specialty testing to get to the root cause of the illness. To conclude that a diagnosis, in this case JIA that is like another common diagnosis, JRA, (Juvenile Rheumatoid Arthritis) should be treated with the same medication, should be questioned, especially when no further workup by the rheumatologist was initiated. Why was monitoring not presented as a viable treatment option, as she was already responding to dietary changes by the first visit to the rheumatologist? Why instead were parents scared into compliance with drug therapy as their only option, with reports of possible permanent joint damage cited as a consequence of not taking the injection at their first visit.

Jenna presented with a similar diagnosis of idiopathic juvenile arthritis. She was nine years of age when she developed severe, progressive pain and stiffness in her wrists, knees and ankles to the point that she was unable to run or play sports. Jenna originally saw an orthopedic doctor who then referred her to a rheumatologist for her symptoms. Basic lab workup was done which was normal. Enbrel, an immunosuppressant, was prescribed to calm the joint inflammation with the agreement that she would need to commit to injections for one full year before stopping them to ensure she stays in remission. That's it – the extent of her workup – your joints are inflamed, and we will calm them down with this drug for one year before entertaining any other treatment plan or workup. Does this make common sense? Of course, mom did not like this treatment plan and sought an integrative approach to her daughter's arthritis. The results of a comprehensive workup done at my office included low Omega 3 essential fatty acids, low amino acids, including low glycine (likely associated with high glyphosate exposures blocking the glycine receptor), high oxidative stress markers, and gluten sensitivities. Just starting her on an anti-inflammatory diet, starting omega 3 EFA, offering probiotics and glutathione helped decrease her joint pains tremendously. Again, why drugs first and long commitments to therapy before investigating the root cause of the arthritis in the first place. Scare tactics were used on both children's parents instead, to evoke compliance with an aggressive solution to prevent further "joint destruction." Methotrexate and Enbrel were Band-aids to the inflammatory response, but at what cost to the patient regarding serious potential acute and future side effects.

So many parents are desperate for their kids to be well and take them to multiple specialists on this quest, but the providers often do not look past the symptoms, and they just prescribe a medication to treat the symptoms or worse than that, tell the parent it is just normal, and they should grow out of it. They do not look past those confining walls of their own construct, to think out of the box and truly improve the health of these children. Although double blinded placebo-controlled studies are great, we do not have time to wait on a study to start getting these kids what they need now. They need better nutrition and less toxic exposures of every kind, period. They need sound medical advice based on common sense not on protocol-driven models of disease management.

Medical science is imprecise, and research is imperfect, but medicine is always evolving, not stagnant. In my 29+ years of being a physician, I have seen the pendulum of recommendations swing wildly from one direction to the other based on "new research." I saw babies placed in bassinets on their bellies in the newborn nursery at Parkland Hospital during my residency, and then overnight the recommendations changed after research showed an increased risk of sudden infant death syndrome with babies laid prone. So, all the babies were then placed on their backs. That said, I have also known of babies who have been tightly swaddled, placed on their back to sleep and have vomited, aspirated and died, and 2-month-old babies who received their first set of vaccinations and within hours were found dead in their crib lying on their back.

I have seen the recommendations for reflux change dramatically in infants. Pediatricians latched on to the antacid, proton pump inhibitor bandwagon for all those fussy, "spitty," "colicky" infants and tired parents having many sleepless nights. Even if the baby did not spit up, they were diagnosed with "silent reflux" and prescribed these antacids just to appease the parents. Years later the American Academy of Pediatrics announced that new research has proven that reflux in kids is not an acid-overproduction problem, and the use of antacids is not indicated, but they continue to be prescribed today despite this research. Necrotizing Enterocolitis, a devastating intestinal disease in premature neonates (especially formula fed) which causes bloody stools and can lead to bowel perforation, sepsis, and even death, was proven to be reduced significantly in the neonatal intensive care unit by the addition of probiotics to the care plan of the neonate. This should have been a widely accepted practice for all NICUs to incorporate probiotic therapy for all neonates, but sadly it was not cost-effective and therefore not implemented as a standard of care protocol.

Uncertainty is common in medicine and there are not many absolutes. With that in mind, we must take a more individualistic approach to providing healthcare, not just following protocols. The one- size-fits-all model of medicine does not work. Functional medicine provides a model for a paradigm shift in healthcare, one that relies on current scientific discoveries paired with an understanding of biochemical individuality and a patient-centered healthcare model. (Vasquez et al., 2010). It is not a prescription that can be tested in a simple random double blinded placebo-controlled study, nor is it a clinical algorithm directing that each patient with condition X is treated with a clearly defined therapy. New advances and theories are gradually embraced, and once they gain acceptance, they become part of normal science. They form the basis for shared beliefs and theories.

Challenging the "standard of care" by replacing it with less recognized or less accepted natural approaches is difficult. Often the natural remedies are not put through the rigorous scientific research as drugs are, so they do not make it on to protocols of "standard of care." On the other hand, drugs are often introduced to the market and later recalled after several months or years, when accumulated anecdotal evidence of harm becomes too significant to overlook. Functional/integrative medicine, in my opinion, is "superior care," as it provides a more comprehensive look at healing rather than just a standard managed care approach to an illness or disease state.

Cochrane reviews are available as systematic reviews of primary research and provide evidence-based healthcare policy statements found in the Cochrane Library. A newer tool embraced by Integrative Medicine practitioners is the Strength of Recommendation Taxonomy (SORT) which is a new grading system that rates the quality, quantity, and consistency of evidence and the strength of recommendations based on a body of evidence. It emphasizes the use of patient-oriented outcomes. Evidence ratings are A-B-C from strongest to weakest evidence, and potential for harm 3-2-1 from highest to lowest. So, an A-1 rating is best, but a C-3 rating is the worst. This tool has been helpful for evaluating natural and medicinal approaches to chronic disease management, specifically as it weights evidence for different therapies, herbal remedies, acupuncture, vitamin/mineral supplementation, etc. This concept was discussed extensively in *Integrative Medicine* (Rakel, 2018), the only textbook I ever read cover to cover twice!

It is unbelievable to me that current new "standard" treatments for eczema now include using Gabapentin, usually used for neuropathy, as off label indication for itching unresponsive to antihistamines. Tacrolimus, Pimecrolimus, and Crisaborole used topically, Methotrexate and Dupixent injectables, and Azathioprim, and Cyclosporin taken orally are just a few of the immunosuppressants used to *control* eczema symptoms

(Lipman et al., 2021). Listed side effects, both common and severe, are disturbing (Drugs.com). Side effects of Gabapentin in children include aggressive behavior, anxiety, concentration problems, changes in school performance, crying, depression, hyperactivity, increase in body movements, mood swings, emotional hyper-reactivity, and restlessness. Listed side effects of any of the immunosuppressants whether topical, oral or injectable are increased risk of serious infections and malignancies that may lead to hospitalization and death. As the latest tools in the western medicine toolbox, they are improving the appearance of eczema for a time, but at what future cost to the health of the child? Going back to "primum non nocere," first do no harm, initiating a therapy that causes a high potential for harm should arguably be a last resort in patient care. A systematic, comprehensive integrative approach should be utilized as the "new standard," using tools such as SORT in evaluating the safest approach to treatment protocols.

4

Principles to Live By

"The doctor of the future will give no medicine but will instruct his patients in the care of the human frame, in diet and in the cause and prevention of disease."

Thomas Edison

Over the years I have adapted my way of practicing medicine, not because of some new protocol or the latest drug released to manage some disease, but through my inner sense of what is right for healing a child as best I can. I offer advice for every aspect of their healthcare – choosing supplements, directing them on healthy food choices, discussing immune support for illnesses, discussing normal development, and referring to a team of integrative colleagues as needed for various issues.

I have drawn upon many modalities to guide my current practice including the Institute of Functional Medicine certification courses, also study of Naturopathic, Chiropractic, Ayurvedic, Homeopathic and Integrative Medicine. Here is a snapshot of what these professions can provide for your health journey.

Naturopathic medicine is based on six principles (Snider & Zeff, 2019):

- First, do no harm (*primum non nocere*).
- Nature has healing powers (*vis medicatrix naturae*).
- Identify and treat the cause (*tolle causam*).
- Treat the whole person (*tolle totum*).
- The physician is a teacher (*docere*).
- Prevention is the best cure (*preventare*).

What I like best about naturopathy is its commonsense approach to health problems. It builds on a positive mental attitude, healthy lifestyle choices such as exercise, sleep, and good health habits, a health-promoting diet, nutritional supplements, and physical modifications such as breathing, posture, and bodywork.

Homeopathic medicine, founded in 1801 by Samuel Hahnemann, and per the American Institute of Homeopathy, officially recognized under the 1938 Food, Drug, and Cosmetic Act, the 1965 Medicare Act, and the 1987 FDA Compliance Policy Guidelines, as safe, gentle but deep-acting medicines that can be used to treat persons experiencing many kinds of medical conditions, is based on the following principles (Demarque et al., 2007):

- Similar (homeo) suffering (pathos), like treats like
- Minimum dose – lower the dose, the greater the effectiveness
- The body has a desire to be well and when it is not in homeostasis, it exhibits symptoms
- Substance made from plant, mineral or animal origin that has been diluted and potentiated, triggers the same clinical picture in healthy patients as the one presented by the sick patient.
- After dilution and dynamization of a particular substance, a curative reaction is induced in the sick patient.
- Materia Medica is a comprehensive resource for choosing the right homeopathic medicines, dilutions and frequency given.

The controversial issue with homeopathy is the western medicine stance that something so diluted would have any beneficial treatment effect on the body. Homeopathy is often called “pseudoscientific alternative medicine” by the naysayers that just don’t understand energy medicine and area quick to point out not enough evidence in real scientific studies or too small of a sample size in observational studies. In my clinical experience, I've found that homeopathy is both safe and effective for treating acute symptoms. Furthermore, for chronically ill patients who require multiple levels of intervention, homeopathy provides an additional option that can help stabilize and optimize their overall health.

Chiropractic medicine is based on these basic principles (Maltese et al., 2019):

- Chiropractic is a form of complementary and alternative medicine that focuses on the relationship between major body structures, such as skeleton, muscles and nerves, and the patient’s health.
- The founder of chiropractic, David Daniel Palmer, called it “a science of healing without drugs.”
- The body has a powerful innate ability to heal itself if given proper support.
- The brain controls body functions through the nervous system.

- Spinal malalignments interfere with the nervous system and can result in lower resistance to disease and many different conditions of suboptimal health.
- Normalizing the relationship between body structure and function can help the body heal.

I like to use the analogy of a garden hose. If the hose is kinked, the water will not flow. The same is true with the electrical energy of your nervous system. I refer to and collaborate care with chiropractors for many common medical complaints such as chronic headaches, constipation, gastroesophageal reflux and sports-related injuries including concussions. I have found that working with chiropractors has led to more speedy recoveries for my patients from any of their presenting problems. As for my extensively fused back and neck, I rely on my chiropractors to keep my moving parts fluid to optimize my function and to avoid pain. I just wish I knew them prior to so many fusion surgeries.

Ayurvedic medicine is based on these basic principles (Jaiswal & Williams, 2017):

- Health and wellness depend on a delicate balance between mind, body and spirit.
- Every person is made up of 5 basic elements found in the universe: space, air, fire, water and earth. These combine in the body to form three life forces or energies called doshas. They control how your

body works. Vata (space & fire), Pitta (fire & water), and Kapha (water & earth)

- Everyone inherits a unique mix of the three doshas with one usually being dominant. Each one controls a body's function. Illness/health issues that develop are linked to imbalances of your doshas.

I do not pretend to be well versed in Ayurvedic medicine, but I do have respect for this modality of healing in the Indian culture. That said, let me tell you about Ananya. She presented to my office with rapid, unexplained hair loss over the course of just a few weeks. She had already seen three different dermatologists and was given three different treatment plans for her alopecia including oral steroids and scalp injections. Parents were not convinced that the treatments suggested were right for her. She was a highly driven, overachiever, often staying up late into the night to finish her studies and learn her lines for a musical she was in. Ananya's thyroid labs were normal and nutrient testing only showed low B vitamins, likely due to chronic stress. I placed her on adrenal support supplements and plant-based vitamins which did help her overall health and energy tremendously. However, the main intervention that made her well was going back to her mother country for one month to receive total care through an Ayurvedic medicine practitioner and learning how to just be still and restore balance to her body. Her hair and her health were fully restored with nutrient support supplements and rest, not with any aggressive steroid injections. The right questions had to be asked to get the right answers and the right treatment plan!

Holistic Dentistry/Airway Management, the newest tool in my toolbox of help for optimizing kids' health. "Improper oral habits can interfere not only with the position of the teeth, but especially with the normal skeletal growth pattern" (Grippaudo et al., 2016). Some basic principles include:

- Mouth breathing causes narrowing of the jaw, teeth crowding and facial narrowing.
- The tongue should always rest on the roof of the mouth and when it doesn't, it causes incorrect swallowing patterns.
- Poor muscle tone of lips and cheeks can also cause dysfunctional swallowing and difficulty sealing the lips. These habits can cause lower teeth crowding and restricted forward jaw growth.
- Lip ties and tongue ties are early clues for impaired mouth anatomy and function.

These findings can lead to sleep disordered breathing and can result in a plethora of health problems including obstructive sleep apnea, hypertrophy of tonsils and adenoids, crowding of teeth, crossbite, and snoring, just to name a few (Davidson, 2022; Gianoni-Capenakas et al., 2020).

Not only do structural issues contribute to airway problems, but inadequate nutrition does as well. Weston A. Price, a Canadian-born dentist and founder of the Weston A. Price Foundation, observed dental decay and physical degeneration in groups of people from all over the world that adopted a more processed food diet (Price, 2009). He documented the healthiest groups of people ate indigenous foods in their culture versus those that abandoned their nutrient rich foods for the modern diet that included white sugar, white flours, refined vegetable oils and canned foods. He observed in just a very short time the perfect dental arches, minimal tooth decay and good health of these people degenerated to deformed jaw structures, crowded and crooked teeth and severe dental caries along with the deterioration of overall health status for those who had moved to a more processed nutrient poor diet.

I would never have even thought about the impact of mouth breathing and snoring as a cause of bed wetting, attention deficit disorder, anxiety, depression, chronic fatigue, cardiovascular disease, headaches and even obesity, had it not been through discussions with my holistic dentist colleagues! Now with my exams on children, I am even more aware of physical findings such as upper lip ties, tongue-ties, tongue position, dental crowding, high arched palates, retrograde lower jaws, mouth breathing, etc. I refer to holistic dentists for early intervention that can be very impactful in preventing chronic health conditions in the future.

Let me tell you about Remi, a perfect example of why it is essential to listen to the patient's entire evolving story in order to develop a comprehensive and transformative solution for their health issues. Remi was partially vaccinated on a slow schedule through 18 months of age. During that time, she developed eczema, keratosis pilaris and had bouts of recurrent abdominal pain that was completely resolved after a gluten free and dairy free diet was initiated, based on results of food sensitivity testing. As she got older, it was obvious that she also had a sensory processing disorder manifesting as behavioral outbursts and extreme tantrums, ultimately requiring occupational therapy. She struggled with frequent night awakenings, night terrors, bedtime anxiety, and bedwetting. Delving deeper into her concerns involved labs that confirmed B complex deficiencies, essential fatty acid deficiencies, yeast and bacterial dysbiosis, high need for glutathione, elevated oxidative markers, environmental toxin metabolites, and positive neuroinflammation markers. Her treatment plan based on the 7Rs of healing included supplementing plant-based antioxidants, probiotics, and glutathione which improved her to another level of health, but did not fully resolve her poor sleep and anxiety. Remi had a history of snoring and enlarged tonsils. An ENT evaluated her and recommended a trial of nasal steroids, while another suggested scheduling surgery to remove her tonsils and adenoids. The nasal steroid trial was ineffective, and her mother declined the surgical option. She was seen instead by a holistic dentist. Evaluation concluded that Remi had a restricted airway which was addressed through myofunctional therapy and an oral appliance specifically designed to tackle the anatomical causes of the airway restriction. At her six-year well visit, mom was elated to report that Remi was like a new child! She no longer experienced night terrors and bedtime anxiety, and her behavioral outbursts dramatically improved. She experienced full recovery not just by one intervention, supplement or dietary modification. A comprehensive, integrative approach was needed to address all her symptoms, with an emphasis on identifying and treating the root cause.

I believe I am most successful in leading people to wellness because of my ability to truly listen to their stories. I draw upon western and eastern medicine simultaneously, whatever seems most needed for that individual patient. I use my experience and insight to guide me. No single approach has all the answers, especially when treating chronic diseases. This balanced approach is what integrative medicine is all about.

Traditional medicine is great at saving lives, but it does not address the wellness aspect of patient care very well.

Traditional medicine looks toward a diagnosis and medication or procedure, or even surgery to "fix the problem." It is the "pill for every ill," Band-Aid-fix approach to disease management. Integrative medicine looks at the subtle signs your body gives you regarding a disruption in function, making it easier to start a treatment plan at this point instead of waiting for a full-blown disease to occur.

Frankly this concept is foreign to most traditional medicine doctors, so they do not embrace it and do not wish to learn about it, citing the "evidence-based medicine" argument. Well, studies take a long time to get published and are often driven by the pharmaceutical companies. I think common sense medicine is a valid approach. Good nutrition just makes sense, and you do not need to cite a study to prove it.

I believe traditional-minded physicians are threatened by this integrative medicine movement because they struggle to understand it. It was just not part of our education. Those of us who consider ourselves "integrative" often have personal stories we can cite that led to our "enlightenment" and new-found passion for a more "holistic, integrative" approach. My conversion was after my own experience as a patient going through nine spinal surgeries and breast cancer. My whole idea of medicine changed from the compartmentalized model of medicine to a more wellness oriented, holistic approach after this experience. I was no closer to "well" after any of my surgeries or breast cancer treatment. To the contrary, my body was ravaged with chemotherapy drugs, oxidative stress, free radical damage to all my organs, and was dangerously nutritionally depleted after my treatments. It has taken years of detoxification, nutritional supplements and whole food nutrition to bring my body back to real health. Breaking free from the "victim mentality" to embracing a "take-charge-of-your-health" mentality" is the first step to "living out of the box!" I know I am on the right track as an integrative medicine practitioner when I have treated eczema, asthma, ADHD, autism, allergies, autoimmune disorders, and many more "diseases" holistically with phenomenal results. I never had this same level of success in treatment, nor the same personal satisfaction in the first ten years I spent managing illness in the traditional medicine model, as I have in the last nineteen years taking a holistic, integrative medicine approach to medical problems.

Let me tell you about Mia. She was literally rolled into my office in a wheelchair for an initial consultation, surrounded by her extended family who were laying hands on her shoulders and mine, praying for me to help heal their chronically ill teenager. She had a 3-month history of progressive weakness and fatigue culminating in being wheelchair-bound due to being unable to walk after receiving the HPV vaccine. Before seeing me, she had already been seen by a rheumatologist and was prescribed oral steroids, and an infectious disease specialist who had already done labs which were all essentially "negative." She had also been seen by a gastroenterologist due to a long history of cyclical vomiting and constipation and was being treated with Zofran, as well as years of daily MiraLAX (polyethylene glycol). She had a history of seasonal allergies and asthma as well as secondary pneumonias and recurrent ER visits for exacerbations. She was treated with multiple rounds of antibiotics, steroids and bronchodilators. Mom was fed up with the system and all the specialists and decided to seek a more holistic approach to her child's symptoms. I again started with the "Cycle of Illness" and "7 R's Healing Program" concept. I told her story back to her in such a way that it all made sense. This was a teenager with a terrible diet, long history of medication use, and constipation. I went to work with labs including food sensitivity testing, nutrient testing and autoimmune markers. She showed high corn and wheat sensitivities, B complex deficiencies, low Vitamin D, yeast and bacterial dysbiosis, low Omega 3 essential fatty acids, neuroinflammation and high heavy metals and positive antinuclear antibodies. I put her on a gluten-free, corn-free diet and started her on a plant-based multivitamin and omega 3 EFA. In just 4 weeks, Mia was walking again, no longer needing a wheelchair! Of course, the family thought it was nothing short of a miracle. At her 3-month follow-up she felt great and continued with the treatment plan. However, 1-1/2 years later Mia developed numbness in her fingers and hair loss that caused her to revisit her health issues with more labs. She had increased antinuclear antibody markers, low Vit D, elevated Thyroid Stimulating Hormone (TSH), low free T4 and positive thyroid peroxidase antibodies (TPO). Mia's ultimate diagnosis was ASIA syndrome – Autoimmune/Inflammatory Syndrome Induced by Adjuvants and Hashimoto's Thyroiditis. According to Watad et al. (2017), adjuvants which are used purposely to enhance the immune response to vaccine, "might also trigger undesired autoimmune reactions," thus questioning their safety. ASIA syndrome has been shown to occur most after HPV, HBV, and seasonal influenza vaccines. The authors discuss developing autoimmune diseases as an adverse effect of the vaccine can be both due to its HPV virus-like particles, which have potent immune-stimulatory properties and due to the presence of aluminum as an adjuvant in the vaccine. Adjuvants can increase, intensify, and prolong antigen-specific immune response of the vaccines, and that "genetically predisposed patients are more likely to exhibit late manifestations and are in a higher risk of developing ASIA syndrome." The article goes on to conclude, "physicians must be mindful that thyroiditis and other thyroid disorders can be induced by diverse adjuvants and therefore to reconsider non-essential vaccination in genetically predisposed individuals for autoimmune diseases." Mia continues to monitor her autoimmune markers, and as best she can, follows a hypoallergenic, autoimmune-paleo diet to keep her in remission from her autoimmune disease.

I believe practicing doctors should have required ongoing exposure and training on integrative medicine approaches to treatment, just as we are required yearly ethics and standard medical education for our specialty. Our kids are our future. I want to do everything in my power to guide parents to raise the healthiest children they can, and that means sound nutrition must be at the foundation. In our highly toxic world with over-processed, nutrient depleted foods, it has become a challenge for parents to accomplish this on their own. Healthy nutrition and lifestyle as well as preventative healthcare should be the focus of every pediatric practice. It is so much easier to prevent disease than it is to treat it once fully manifested. Prevention messages in pediatrics focus mostly on being up to date on vaccinations, developmental screening for early interventional therapy, growth, hearing and vision, screening for substance abuse, anxiety and depression. It is time for all pediatricians to broaden their definition of "health care and well check-up visits.

5

Inspiration for Transformation

"Medicine is a science of uncertainty and an art of probability."

Sir William Osler

Changing to a different view of healthcare requires a paradigm shift in thinking. (Vasquez et al., 2010). Both Functional and Integrative medicine focus on a patient-centered approach that encourages taking personal responsibility for your health and well-being. I encourage my colleagues to go beyond being a mere healthcare technician and become a healer of the whole person. The patients I take care of and their families, hunger for information and choice more than a prescription. The time when healthcare providers were unquestioned authorities in white coats is long over. We must learn to work collaboratively with our patients in a role that is more like mentoring, counseling and guiding them towards wellness. The practitioner-centered care model where the practitioner is an unquestioned authority figure is being replaced by a patient-centered self-care model. I welcome the hard questions posed to me by the families I care for. I welcome the internet research they present to me as they actively search for their own answers. My patients often talk to me about how expensive medications are and their fear of side effects, so they are very open to alternatives therapies such as dietary modifications, vitamins, minerals, herbal and homeopathic remedies that can help their condition safely and, in most cases, less expensively. Having safe and effective choices provided by a knowledgeable healthcare provider is key. Some of my patients prefer natural, some conventional therapies, but most importantly I meet the family where they are and provide a wide range of choices. In my experience, parents are desperate for information with which they can be empowered to transform the health of their family. They are tired of being told "party-line," "standard of care protocol" answers to their questions and leaving with prescriptions to just manage their complaints.

Being healthy is a choice and takes hard work. Being real with my families and understanding the pitfalls to living a healthy lifestyle, makes me an effective practitioner. I often tell parents that if they make just one healthier choice today than they did yesterday, they will be healthier tomorrow than they are today. Lao Tsu, an ancient Chinese philosopher once said, "A journey of a thousand miles begins with one step." Curing a disease primarily addresses physical health. Healing someone involves integrating body, mind, and spirit approaches to achieve wholeness. Henry David Thoreau once said "Nature is doing her best each moment to make us well. She exists for no other end. Do not resist. With the least inclination to be well, we should not be sick." The very thing that is often ignored by doctors in the healing process is the very thing I utilize the most to guide someone to wellness – nutrition! I have taken care of so many very seriously ill children with significant medical conditions throughout the years including cancer, severe eczema and failure to thrive, autoimmune disease, asthma, ASD, just to name a few. I may not be able to make these disease states go away, but I can certainly do all I can to optimize their health and healing in the process. Many of these children are on long term medications that are raking havoc on their immune system and gut flora. Others must have multiple surgeries for their condition, creating oxidative stress and free radical damage in the process. The body is an intricate web of connections and what we do to one organ system has far reaching consequences potentially good or bad on the rest of the body. Knowing this principle allows me to take a step back and see potential nutritional needs for each child's complex medical issues. Although the details of each child's development of a "disease state" are unique, the process of optimizing their healing is the same, and it starts with utilizing the "Cycle of Illness" and "7Rs of Healing" approach, laying the foundation for the body to essentially push the "reset button." I do not promise to cure anyone. My job as a healer is to provide tools for families to give their children the best chance to thrive. As Hippocrates said long ago, "Let food be thy medicine and medicine be thy food." The practice of medicine used to be such an art of healing. Physicians have been known to be some of the most creative, "out of the box" thinkers. Unfortunately, today I see the idealistic, energetic medical student being indoctrinated into a corporate-compliance model of healthcare that is more of a protocol driven managed care system where he is nothing but a technician or peddler of pharmaceutical drugs. Our patients deserve more than that.

Let me tell you about Caleb. He has had severe eczema, asthma, and allergies his whole life. He suffers all year round with seasonal flares. He sees an allergist for his IgE food and environmental allergies who manages his symptoms with prescription antihistamines and nasal steroids and recently started a regimen of allergy shots. Caleb also sees a pulmonologist for his asthma. He is often in the moderate risk zone for his symptoms and was hospitalized for severe asthma once around the age of three. He has been to the ER on average once or twice a year. Mom admits she has not found a pattern in his flare ups and cannot determine if his flare ups occur seasonally or after eating a certain food. Mom has noticed that when he is sick his breathing is almost always labored. His symptoms have been managed with prescription medications including inhaled or oral steroids, bronchodilators, and immune modulator medications on a regular, almost daily basis. Asthma has been an ongoing battle for Caleb, and according to mom it is the scariest of his diagnoses, especially when it cannot be controlled even with all his medications. His eczema is the worst visible diagnosis, mainly because it never clears. His skin is always red, and irritated, and if the eczema improves with medications, it does not last long, maybe a couple of days. Mom reports that it is so hard for her to watch her child itch and scratch uncontrollably to the point of making his skin bleed. The minute his medications wear off, he reverses the progress through his scratching. He has been managed by a dermatologist with hydroxyzine and high potency steroid ointments for his itching, Aquaphor topically as his moisturizer, bleach baths about once a week to prevent bacterial overgrowth on his skin, and wet dressings when his skin is severely cracked and inflamed. He has had several skin infections due to his open sores, which have been managed with multiple antibiotics. Like Caleb's asthma medication regimens, mom also admitted to me at his first visit that she struggles to comply with his eczema protocols. She felt like she had failed her son because she could not do everything perfectly to get him better. Mom also voiced her concerns regarding the side effects of his steroid inhalers and topical and oral steroids, as her son is very small for age. Mom had read that steroids may stunt growth but was reassured by the specialists and previous primary care provider that the side effects were minimal.

Mom came to my office desperate for answers and a different approach to leading her son back to wellness, not just Band-Aid fixing his symptoms. Mom reported that Caleb is a very active, normal 7-year-old. He is very tough and cooperative when it comes to administering his medications and taking his conditions in stride. He wants to play all the sports and ride dirt-bikes with his cousins, but so much of his activities are limited due to parents' fears that his asthma or eczema will flare. Mom wanted what every parent desires, to give her son the gift of health, free of pain and medications, free to live his life to the fullest. So, I went to work. I reiterated his progression to chronic disease demonstrated in "The Cycle of Illness" and how seemingly unrelated diagnoses are all interconnected. I told his story back to mom using this visual. It was such a light bulb moment for her, and something that had never been discussed or even brought up by any of her specialists. I discussed dysbiosis, leading to a state of malabsorption and the development of food sensitivities, which can predictably result in nutrient depletion and thus lead to the development of many chronic diseases including eczema, asthma, allergies, neurocognitive and neurobehavioral problems, and weakened immune system in general. I discussed lab testing first to determine food and respiratory allergies and food sensitivities, checked for anemia and checked his Vitamin D level. I placed him on a hypoallergenic diet – no dairy, soy, egg, wheat, nuts, corn, and put him on high dose probiotic 25 billion cfu daily. I stopped the bleach baths, gave him Mupirocin ointment for cracked skin and to use in nostrils three times weekly to treat staph colonization, and instructed him to use some hypoallergenic creams and oils on his skin, and awaited lab results.

One month later during his lab review, Caleb was smiling ear to ear, was less itchy, more comfortable, still had dark circles under his eyes and was very thin for age, 66% height, 39% for weight. As predicted, Caleb was sensitive to all the inflammatory foods he was asked to cut out. His skin was much improved, clearing centrally, less red and irritated, but still had cracking in places on his extremities. I placed him on a medical food protein powder, L-glutamine, omega 3 essential fatty acids, digestive enzymes with each meal and saw him 3 weeks later. At that time, mom reported a mild asthma attack after accidentally eating chocolate covered nuts – caused initially an eczema flare, then wheezing a day later. Mom treated Caleb with Albuterol and felt he responded quickly. On exam, Caleb's skin was remarkably clearer with only one patch of redness on his cheek and a clear but dry trunk. His extremities showed only cracks on his hands and feet, very dry, but no rash! I continued the mupirocin ointment to the deep cracks to prevent invasion of staph bacteria, continued topical nourishing skin oils as well as added other healthy fats to his diet such as olive oil, avocado oil and flax seed oil. I continued his current supplements. He even asked if he could take the protein shake more than once a day. His height was 67% and weight increased to 46%. I discussed with Caleb and mom that these diet restrictions are not for forever. I reiterated the 7Rs of healing program and that it may take 3-6 months and sometimes even longer, but at the other end, most kids are significantly better from whatever the chronic state of ill health they were in.

The reason the specialists could not make any progress in curing Caleb was that they were too focused on managing the symptoms. The parent was told that his eczema and asthma were chronic, incurable diseases and were best to be managed throughout his lifetime. As medical doctors we are trained to diagnose and treat or manage, not necessarily to cure. Especially with chronic disease, the medical system just does not have the tools to come up with a comprehensive treatment plan such as this that is nutrition-based and focuses on the cure. As you can see, in just 2 months we took a failure to thrive child with severe allergies, got him off medications, off allergy shots, and on true solid ground nutritionally with supplementation and an anti-inflammatory diet. He has a long way to go but is well on his way to optimal health, but I know he is determined enough to get there.

This case reflects a concept that is so prevalent in medicine, *anchoring bias* and *diagnosis momentum.* "Cognitive biases in clinical practice have a significant impact on care, often in negative ways" (Doherty & Carroll, 2020). First, *anchoring bias* is the tendency to draw conclusions too early in the presentation based on initial impressions despite new information. The second pitfall, *diagnosis momentum*, is a phenomenon whereby once diagnostic labels are attached to patients they just "stick" and are never removed. Interestingly, I stumbled onto these terms while completing my continual medical education requirement for my medical license ethics. I see many "problem lists" and "diagnosis summaries" as part of new patient records and to me, they tell a story. The story is about a child who started down a path of illness – recurrent respiratory infections, ear infections, then the development of allergies, asthma, developmental delays, you name it. I see the pattern that emerged that got them to that state of ill health. Sadly, to most physicians, this list serves only as a summary of diagnoses and treatments that are considered standard of care. Conventional medicine is not looking to "clean the slate" and get you well. Instead, the goal is more often to have these "unfortunate diagnoses" well managed by the continually increasing list of state-of-the-art medications and procedures. Caleb had a large list of diagnoses that one by one are coming off the description of who he is. With each visit I could see the real child coming out, smiling, at ease, starting to really enjoy life. Losing the labels should be our goal, not creating longer lists to manage.

Let me share another disturbing example patient of anchoring bias and diagnosis momentum. Jason was a 4-year-old sweet mild-mannered child who first came to see me after he had been admitted to a local children's hospital with a seizure. He was observed overnight and had an EEG which showed post seizure slow wave activity and was prescribed Keppra. No further workup was done by the neurologist to investigate the "why" behind the new onset seizure disorder. Mom felt uneasy about starting a seizure medication that she was told he would have to take for 2 years before considering a trial off, so mom sought my help and drove 2 hours to my office for a different approach.

As part of my initial work up, I obtained comprehensive nutrient labs which showed B-complex vitamin, Zinc, Magnesium and Manganese deficiencies, Vitamin D deficiency, methylation impairment, low essential fatty acids, low glutathione, and elevated mercury levels. I placed him on an all-inclusive plant-based vitamin, mineral and amino acid supplement, a multi-strain probiotic, and further detoxification support with glutathione. Multiple follow-ups were done over the next two years without any sign of seizures.

Then at 6 years of age the unthinkable happened, a bizarre, tragic accident that landed him back at the very hospital he was admitted to previously for his seizure disorder. A desperate phone call came in at 2 am from this frantic mom saying her child had been run over by a riding lawnmower and needed to go to surgery right away to reattach his sciatic nerve. Parents were told that he may never walk again and would likely be in the hospital for 6 weeks or more. I remember having a strangely calm conversation with mom in the wee morning hours and told her I knew everything was going to be ok. Things happen randomly or maybe not so randomly as it turned out.

During the intake process to the hospital the nurse reviewed his previous history and commented on making sure Keppra was ordered for his seizure disorder for him to continue during his hospital stay. Mom told the nurse that he was not on any seizure medication and in fact that he was a patient of mine and that he was treated naturally and has never had another seizure. During his hospital stay at one point mom said she had an entire audience of nurses in Jason's room hearing his story about how he was cured of his seizure disorder. Mom even convinced the staff to allow him to take the probiotics, vitamins and glutathione he was on at home to offset the high dose antibiotics, anesthesia and free radical damage that he likely had because of tissue trauma and surgery. Amazingly, Jason also left the hospital walking with the help of a walker just 2-1/2 weeks after the accident, not 6-8 weeks as previously predicted! Several of the staff's eyes were opened to a whole world of healing that did not fit into their neat little protocols and problem lists and they were forever changed and inspired by Jason's spirit and quick recovery in an "out of the box" way.

6

Breaking Free

"Health is not valued until sickness comes."

Thomas Fuller

"Healing is a matter of time, but it is sometimes also a matter of opportunity."

Hippocrates

Just as Moses was divinely commissioned to lead the people out of Egyptian slavery, so too I feel integrative medicine doctors lead their patients out of their own disease enslavement and out of the very system that perpetuates it.

Let me tell you about Henry. He started as a newborn in my practice. He was a term baby born by C-section. Mom started coming to see me initially with her 15-month-old who had chronic ear infections and speech delay. She was frustrated by the continued use of antibiotics without any mention of testing or investigation of the root cause of her child's illness. He was offered standard vaccination schedules and therapies. Fast forward to her new baby, mom wanted a new approach to raising a healthier child. Henry had some initial cradle cap and case of erythema toxicum newborn rash in the newborn nursery but was otherwise healthy appearing at his first checkup. But at 2 months old he started having some mild, dry eczema patches. I recommended topical emollients such as coconut oil and calendula cream, and asked mom to take an omega 3 supplement and a probiotic while breast feeding. He received only a DTaP vaccine at that visit due to the parent's desire for a slower vaccine schedule. He developed congestion and cold symptoms as well as a progressive outbreak of "rashy" eczema spreading down trunk and arms in the three weeks that followed the vaccination. I focused more on mom's diet and asked her to do an elimination diet of top allergens including dairy, soy, eggs, wheat, and peanuts. Mom admitted that she eats a lot of peanut butter and drinks a lot of milk, so I told her to do a trial elimination of both these foods completely, and if the rashy eczema does not resolve, work on further elimination of top allergenic foods. I also recommended Evening Primrose oil rubbed on his skin and to follow up in two weeks at his well checkup.

At his 4-month well visit, mom was frustrated and said nothing seemed to be working to clear his eczema despite the trial elimination diet of all allergenic foods, probiotics and omega 3. I recommended a comprehensive digestive stool analysis to determine whether he was colonized with any yeast or dysbiotic bacteria that may be causing his suspected malabsorption and sensitivities to the foods mom was eating while nursing. Henry was born by Cesarian section which puts him at high risk for abnormal colonization, especially given mom's history of yeast infection and antibiotic exposure at delivery. I prescribed a topical steroid as a Band-Aid fix to provide relief from his scratching while I figured out the underlying cause of his persistent poorly responsive eczema. My suspicions were correct. Henry's stool analysis showed Blastocystis hominus, Klebsiella, and yeast dysbiosis with inadequate expected E. coli or Bifidobacteria colonization. I treated him with an antibiotic, as well as prebiotic fiber and a multi-strain probiotic. He also had signs of gut inflammation and malabsorption of carbohydrates and short chain fatty acids. No wonder he could not get well.

At his 9-month checkup he continued to avoid wheat and dairy in his diet as well as in mom's while still nursing. Mom reported that his eczema had completely cleared while on prebiotic fiber and probiotics and after the prescription antibiotic, but when the supplements were discontinued for repeat stool testing, his eczema patches returned, just dry patches, not "rashy" eczema as before. At his 1-year checkup mom reported that his eczema was completely clear until going on vacation and not taking prebiotic fiber and probiotic supplements. He had some rough skin on his trunk, but no rashes. I added L-glutamine, collagen, and rotating healthy oils to his diet. Mom was amazed that these were the missing links to his healing. He had a severe episode of croup at 17 months and a few minor colds treated with natural remedies, but other than that, he was finally healed. Skip forward to the 2-year checkup, I see a healthy happy child with no eczema or signs of allergies. Mom was able to reintroduce all the foods he was previously sensitive to. She decided to resume vaccines at this point, so he received the DTaP vaccine. This was only his second vaccine by parent choice due to his chronic health issues. He promptly developed a softball sized swelling at the injection site which was very itchy and red and had to be treated with

Epsom salt baths, bentonite clay packs, and antihistamines to fully resolve.

Although his course has been rough, the problems were isolated at their roots and dealt with in a custom care way, always having in mind restoration of health and balanced immune system. Mom is a proud believer in the power of integrative medicine techniques. But she also says that even today, when she tells other doctors about the success they have had with alternative/integrative medicine techniques, they brush her off and seem uninterested in what was done to heal him. Mom says we are an "answer to our prayers" and the reason she still drives 2 hours one way to come to well-visits!

Ariana is a 3-year-old with a history of chronic sinus infections. At the first visit to my office, mom disclosed a printout of the 18 courses of antibiotics she had been prescribed for repeated diagnosis of otitis and sinusitis by the urgent care and primary care physician office over a one-year time span. Mom said she was frustrated and was done with this approach to managing her child's symptoms. No allergy testing or any other testing had been offered by the other doctors, despite mom requesting it. She knew something was wrong but had nowhere to turn and no one was listening to her pleas for help. She presented with other symptoms to our office including chronic, recurrent diarrhea and vomiting. She had a significant past medical history of having a normal vaginal birth but had E coli sepsis and meningitis at 10 days of age which required treatment with 2 weeks of intravenous antibiotics. She had multiple antibiotic courses for recurrent ear infections, which eventually led to pressure equalizing tube placement and adenoidectomy at 20 months of age. She also had moderate to severe eczema that was treated with topical steroids and lotions. More recently she has developed recurrent wheezing requiring inhaler therapy. Basically, this child's first 2 years of life were miserable for this family, filled with sleepless, fussy nights, urgent care and specialist visits, surgery for ear tubes, and seemingly endless prescriptions.

Mom was desperate for a new approach and was frustrated by the system and needed to know a way out and a new set of truths. I obtained a comprehensive stool analysis to investigate specific dysbiosis markers, IgG food sensitivity and IgE food and respiratory allergy testing, along with CBC, Comprehensive metabolic panel, and immunoglobulin profile due to recurrent illnesses requiring antibiotic intervention. I again discussed the "Cycle of Illness" and "7Rs of healing" as a framework for understanding how Ariana got so sick and to outline the steps needed to achieve true healing (Recognize, Re-inoculate, Remove, Replace, Repair and Rebalance and Recover). I discussed starting with an elimination diet of the most common inflammatory foods, multivitamin supplementation and probiotics, to start after testing was obtained. Labs revealed significant dysbiosis, predictable with the number of antibiotic courses she had in the past. She also had a high dog dander allergy and moderate soy, dairy, and flax sensitivity. Ariana remained on the anti-inflammatory diet, avoiding dairy, soy and most gluten and returned in 3 months smiling contagiously. She reported that since she started the healing program her daughter has not had any sinus related issues, her eczema completely cleared up, her abdominal pain resolved, and her daughter's energy soared.

Here is a mom who, in the past, relied heavily on the medical system and felt it was just inevitable for her daughter to need antibiotics every month. With each visit I could see mom breaking free from the grip the system had on her, breaking free of that rigid box she was in. I saw new hope and determination and a new sense of confidence build up in mom as she stepped out in faith and trusted in another way. Mom saw how powerful restoring balance to her digestive tract by taking probiotics and avoiding a few inflammatory foods could positively affect her health. She was seeing the light shining into that rigid box. She was becoming the "mama warrior" shouting from outside of the box, telling everyone about the transformation in her beliefs and in her child's health.

Then the unthinkable happened. The family traveled to a small town in the Midwest during harvest season. With Ariana's history of food sensitivities, she had been on a very clean diet for the last year, but on the trip, mom said the whole family had to eat foods they were not used to, lots of gluten and dairy containing meals, processed foods, etc. Ariana started showing sinus symptoms almost immediately. Then things took a turn for the worse. Ariana had a severe, life-threatening asthma attack while she was eating pizza for dinner and developed progressive shortness of breath and wheezing. She was rushed to a local hospital and was found to have oxygen saturation in the 80's and was given repeated nebulizer treatments to improve her breathing. The doctors gave her IV and oral steroids, very high dose antibiotics Rocephin and Azithromycin for suspected pneumonia. Mom says she felt at the mercy of the treating physicians and did not have any say in treatment. She felt they were not listening to her regarding the possible allergic component of her abrupt onset of wheezing. I sat there in the exam room and listened to this nightmare experience and the sheer rigid protocol-based standard of care medicine that was being administered to this child. Yes, it was lifesaving, but why more antibiotics? Mom certainly questioned this but felt afraid to resist these "in the box" thinking doctors who were trying to save her daughter's life. We discussed the likely scenario that led to her respiratory compromise and the need for hospitalization. I believe it probably started with her exposure over several days to the pro-inflammatory diet she had been avoiding for the last year as well as staying in an old farmhouse with dog dander to which she is allergic, and exposure to the corn crops being harvested. All these factors contributed to a severe asthma attack within days of arrival. Although antibiotics are important for serious infections, the last thing this child needed, given her history, was more antibiotics thrust upon her for an allergy related event. Just weeks after this episode, she had more of a viral induced wheezing episode preceded by a low-grade fever and runny nose. It would have been easy to just try another antibiotic for presumed "bronchitis", after all, she had had a week of viral symptoms, but instead we focused on a comprehensive history and did a lab test that confirmed the diagnosis of RSV (respiratory syncytial virus) bronchiolitis that did not require antibiotic therapy. As part of the Cycle of Illness discussed earlier, Ariana was certainly experiencing a weakened immune system causing her to be more susceptible to picking up any virus. We refocused again on the 7Rs healing program, especially after recent antibiotic exposure. Mom got her back on track with the healing anti-inflammatory diet, multivitamins, probiotics, omega 3 essential fatty acids, Vitamin D and other immune support homeopathic and herbal remedies to get her well again.

Through all these illnesses, Ariana's parents became more and more informed and empowered to take charge of their whole family's health by learning about natural ways to approach medical problems, which ultimately gave them hope of true wellness and allowed them to break free from the victim mentality that had been so deeply rooted in years past.

7

Following Blindly – Really?

"Learn from yesterday, live for today, hope for tomorrow. The important thing is not to stop questioning."

Albert Einstein

"The preservation of health is easier than the cure of the disease."

BJ Palmer, DC

An ever-growing alphabet soup of medical diagnoses has erupted over the years. Acronyms such as POTS, FPIES, ARFIDS, EoE, PANDAS, PANS, SPD, ADHD, ASD, etc. created by conventional medicine specialists have become common terms, but labeling does not make the physician any closer to the root cause and cure, but just offers a special Band-aid with which to manage it.

Let me tell you about Liam. He came to my office as a teenager with a history of uncontrollable motor tics for 7 years prior to seeing me. He had been seen previously by several doctors including neurologists, all of whom wanted to put him on medication for Tourette's syndrome which mom refused and sought my help to get to the root of his problem. Other history uncovered at his first visit to my office included chronic recurrent abdominal pain, recurrent diarrhea and this intrusive movement disorder. On the exam he was significantly overweight, had very disturbing almost continuous chorea-form serpentine-like movements of his shoulders, chest, neck and arms, worse than I have ever seen. He also had extensive keratosis pilaris "KP" otherwise known as "chicken skin" on his arm, face and back. His workup by other doctors was basic but did find he had a fatty liver. No explanation for this was given and no treatment plan suggested except to watch his fat intake and take Clonidine to treat the tic disorder.

I went to work with a comprehensive evaluation of his state of health using the "Cycle of Illness" and "7Rs Healing" program as a guide for the parents to follow. I did food sensitivity testing, comprehensive stool testing and nutrient testing. I found that he had dairy and wheat sensitivities, and elevated markers for PANDAS, an acronym for Pediatric Autoimmune Neuropsychiatric Disorder Associated with Strep throat. He had low levels of Vitamin D3, B-complex vitamins, Zinc, and Selenium, as well as imbalanced essential fatty acids with low Omega 3, normal thyroid and glycemic control testing. I put him on a dairy-free, gluten-free, sugar restricted, minimally processed food diet. I started him on a food-based multivitamin, Vitamin D3, multi-strain probiotic, glutathione, as well as a homeopathic strep remedy. Liam admittedly was a "carboholic" and junk food, highly processed, fast-food consumer previously. He really took ownership of the advice given based on lab results and wanted to get better. He could not even focus on work at school due to the intrusive serpentine movements. Putting it all together for him by pointing out nutrient deficiencies and food sensitivities gave him tangible steps to take to get better. Over the course of one year, his motor tics/abnormal movements were completely resolved, his KP resolved, and he lost 60 pounds just by following a healthy minimally processed food diet, offering detoxification and nutrient support. Repeat labs were taken along the way to fine tune his treatment plan. Testing and retesting are important to help keep the patient and family engaged in the process. I also feel it is important to journal mini triumphs along the way to be able to look back and see progress when it seems like little progress is being made. Remember, your child did not get to this disease state overnight and it takes time to rebalance and repair to recover!

Tic disorders are categorized based on presentation and length of symptomatology (American Psychiatric Association, 2022). Tics are sudden, involuntary movements (motor tic) or uttered sounds (verbal tic) that occur during otherwise normal behavior. Common tics include eye blinking, nose twitching, head jerking or shoulder shrugging.

- Tourette syndrome patients exhibit both motor and vocal tics and have had tic symptoms for at least 1 year.
- Persistent motor or vocal tic disorder patients exhibit either motor or vocal tics and have had tic symptoms for at least 1 year.
- Provisional tic disorder patients can exhibit motor or vocal tics, or both, but have had their symptoms for less than 1 year.

Studies have estimated that 1 in 162 children have Tourette syndrome and many children diagnosed with this disorder also have other behavioral, developmental and mental disorders (Centers for Disease Control and Prevention, 2024). Medication and behavioral therapy are sited to help control or reduce tic frequency and improve quality of life but do not result in remission of the disease itself. The cause of tic disorders is unknown, although speculated to be at least worsened by sleep deprivation and stress.

Now if I were an "in the box" thinker, newly trained healthcare provider, I would take this information at face value and not even blink an eye. However, in my experience dealing with many children in my practice with motor and verbal tics that are now resolved, I respectfully disagree. An underlying multifaceted situation can usually be discovered through a root-cause, functional medicine approach, which has led to the motor/verbal tic symptoms. Sam, for example, is another a teenager in my practice with facial motor tics. He recently had an escalation of his blinking and facial grimacing that prompted his parents to seek my help for possible medication for Tourette's. My comprehensive lab work was essentially normal except for some B complex vitamin and Magnesium deficiencies. I had him undergo a Zyto Balance energy scan in my office that showed acute EMF-driven stressors that may have contributed to his symptoms. This was a teen who could not unplug from his many technical gadgets – ear buds, tablets, phone, smart devices, and TV in his room. Could it have been the cause of his motor tics? I do not know for sure, but what I do know is that he did a trial of Clonidine briefly, used EMF blocking technology to limit his exposure to the electromagnetic frequencies from his gadgets, and his motor tics resolved. At his 3 month follow up checkup, Sam was also able to be weaned off Clonidine without return of his tics. I have found that addressing neuro-inflammation markers, detoxification, and doing a trial elimination diet of inflammatory foods, all have helped reduce symptoms. Once again, getting to the root cause of the "tic disorder" should be the goal of the practitioner, not just prescribing a medication such as Clonidine for the management/control of symptoms.

Let me tell you about Risha, another potential casualty of the western medicine system approach to her condition. She is a 15-month-old toddler who is now fully recovered from eczema in just a few short months under my care. She initially saw me at 9 months of age. She had a history of an ear infection at 3 months of age treated with antibiotics by per previous pediatrician. She had a viral respiratory infection at 4 months of age and within a week of the illness had her standard vaccines. Two days after vaccinations, she had an eczema outbreak on her legs, arms, face and neck. The facial eczema turned into an oozing weepy impetigo superinfection which was again treated with oral antibiotics and topical mupirocin as well as topical steroids and nystatin. She started eating foods at 6 months of age including fruits, vegetables, but also eggs and peanut butter per the new recommendations of early introduction of potentially allergenic foods to prevent food allergies. She developed hives and worsening eczema and was referred to an allergist by per her previous pediatrician. Labs obtained by the allergist showed a class 5 egg white allergy, class 3 peanut and cashew allergy, class 2 cow milk and soy allergy. The allergist said to return to his office for low dose immunotherapy by offering small amounts of these allergenic foods to her in the office with the ability to give her an antihistamine and epinephrine injection if needed for any reaction such as hives, swelling of the lips or respiratory distress! Mom elected to use some common sense instead. She sought an alternative approach to her healthcare which included healing her leaky gut likely caused by the antibiotic exposures and disruption of healthy gut flora, avoiding unnecessary toxins and foreign protein injections with vaccinations, and avoiding allergenic foods. With our integrative medicine healthcare approach, Risha's skin is now soft and smooth- appearing with no rashes. She has not required any life-saving interventions with antihistamines or epinephrine injections and continues a hypoallergenic whole food diet to ensure the best chances of reintroducing these foods after further testing planned at 2 years of age.

I was taught in my medical training to introduce eggs and nuts/nut butters at 1 year of age and shellfish and honey at two years of age as well as introduce foods one at a time.

The new recommendations for early introduction of potentially allergenic foods at 4 months of age do not resonate well with my common sense, nor my old-school training way of thinking. The new way does not necessarily mean a better way. For example, the new puree pouches that have every nut represented in them do not make sense if you hold true to the recommendation of introducing one new food at a time, waiting a few days before trying another food to ensure tolerance. You must ask yourself where the recommendations are coming from and are they based on sound reproducible facts or on flawed research. In my medical school training I learned that statistically, 75% of IgE egg white allergies are resolved by 7 years of age, majority of cow milk allergies by 5 years of age, and soy allergies by 2 years of age. So, if this is the case, then is it a viable option to wait on aggressive intervention? Patients I help with my integrative medical approach think out of the box like I do and want alternative routes of evaluation and treatment that are safe, and not conformist views and protocol-driven approaches to their medical treatment.

8

Ripping off the Band-Aid

"Imagine a world in which medicine was oriented toward healing rather than disease, where doctors believed in the natural healing capacity of human beings and emphasized prevention above treatment. In such a world, doctors and patients would be partners working toward the same ends."

Andrew Weil, MD

Western medicine does not have all the answers and to claim it does is both arrogant and ignorant. The children in the stories presented did not get better with a one-size-fits-all, Band-Aid-fix approach to their health problems. Each child has a unique history that can be retold in a functional medicine way, with the end goal of restoration of their health, not just managing their symptoms. Their recoveries were achieved mostly by attention to nutrition, gut health and detoxification, not by any drug or procedure.

A preventative medicine model must be embraced to prevent the predictable imbalances that lead to an ultimate disease state. The frightening statistics on chronic disease presented are real and disturbing and do not show any favorable turns in the foreseeable future. Envision a bankrupted economy with a growing chronically ill population with not enough facilities or drugs to care for them all. We have already seen glimpses of this reality with antibiotic shortages, ADHD medication shortages and extensive waitlists for therapists and specialty schools for autism and other learning differences. There are not enough facilities to put them in when their parents pass. What are we going to do with the aging autistic and chronically ill population – who is going to take care of them? Raising healthy children into healthy adults should be our goal. "Autism Awareness" month at least brought attention to the fact that we have a problem to address.

Changing to "Autism Acceptance" month implies no action is required and that we are just accepting and embracing autistic children's differences now. What happened to questioning why a perfectly developing child suddenly regressed and started headbanging and lost all verbal and social skills? Where is the curiosity about why the autism rate has increased exponentially without a change in our genetics? Where is the solution? People are suffering. Families are being torn apart emotionally and financially taking care of these kids. I see the lonely battle of families of autistic kids in this rigid "in the box" medical system almost daily, given no hope for a cure – only being told to accept their "differences." I have parents with tears of guilt, tears of helplessness and grief turn to tears of joy and hope in my intake visits as I reframe what they have been through by a different compassionate, caring lens of truth. Why is there a therapy center on almost every corner? What could we have done differently? Is there another option to getting all the vaccines, all at once on the exact same schedule? Frustrated parents ask their pediatrician, "why can't I do a modified schedule? It's my child. What do you mean I will be fired if I do not comply," but it often lands on deaf ears and ends with the statement, "it's just standard of care." How can it be "standard of care" when it differs from state to state and from country to country? If we stop asking any questions, we will not get any answers and we will just become compliant consumers stuffed in the dark ridged box called the healthcare system. It is time to embrace a different set of truths and break free of the establishment constructs that may be keeping you well managed but not any closer to being well.

If there is a risk, you should have a choice. Violating fundamental patients' rights without proper consent is wrong. To force or expect someone to take a drug, surgery, or vaccination without explaining the risk and benefit is absurd. There is no place for any forced procedure without true informed consent. Children have no voice. They rely on wise, informed adults to help with decision making at every level of their care to raise them into healthy adults. Coercion to gain compliance is not acceptable.

I remember a particular Texas Pediatric Society Meeting where a picture of Dr. Sears, author of "The Vaccine Book," was put on the big screen to make an intentional derogatory point about him and his book. Immediate boos and chanting of insulting comments followed in this crowd mentality form. It was so scary what I witnessed in this brainwashed audience. I remember just sinking low in my chair as I cringed and wanted to make myself invisible. I worked hard to become Functional Medicine certified, Integrative Medicine Board certified, Homeopathy certified, and Homeoprophylaxis certified to liberate myself from the ridged "in the box" thinking mindset the western medicine model had to offer, but also as protection from the close-minded doctors that had a narrower view of medicine. As a pioneer of holistic integrative pediatric medicine, I felt alone, threatened, and even at one point called a "quack" by the establishment physicians, but once you know the truth, you cannot go back. I knew there was another way that was being hidden from me by just listening to party-line speakers at these conferences. I sought real science and real medicine to shape my recommendations. Families deserve more than this current medical model. I am not anti-vaccine, but I am pro-choice and pro true informed consent for any intervention especially when it could potentially cause harm. If I have a vaccine hesitant family, I am equipped to offer knowledge about alternative, modified, delayed and selective schedules, spreading vaccines out to suit their comfort level. I can also offer another method of protection without injection, namely homeoprophylaxis for those families that are determined not to do any vaccinations.

Dr. Isaac Golden, a champion in the field of homeopathy, states that Homeo-prophylaxis is a "viable alternative" to injectable vaccinations with 90% effectiveness and without the known toxic side effects listed on the vaccine information forms (Golden, 2010). With over 20 years of solid research, he believes that not every infectious disease is a major threat to a healthy infant. He says that "parents can provide a high level of protection against targeted diseases, without risk, by using an appropriate HP program." He goes on to say that "criticism without facts is the antithesis of the true scientific method, yet it is the response we continually get from pharmaceutical medicine when it comes to HP." He boldly states that those who claim that there is no evidence supporting the effectiveness of HP are clearly wrong and that it is not essential to rely only on randomized clinical trials (RCTs) to provide evidence of effectiveness. Furthermore, Dr. Golden says that "a natural immunization system, where both vaccination and HP were available to parents, would increase the national coverage against targeted infectious diseases and reduce the incidence of some chronic health conditions, especially asthma." Shouldn't this be the goal of every parent and every healthcare provider, to protect without doing harm? It is the job of parents to teach their children about nutrition and healthy choices to set them up for success. It is the job of the healthcare industry to equip families with education and guidance to help them do the same. The goal of the well visit should not be to comply with an aggressive vaccine schedule that continues to grow in number "required." Parents should be given choices and have true informed consent with what they are putting in their child's body. Healthcare providers should be open-minded to alternative ways of treating an illness, not just prescribing a pharmaceutical.

Working with an ever expanding integrative, natural-minded network of healthcare providers has been extremely rewarding to me both personally and professionally. Families are eagerly seeking this type of care for a reason – managed sick care does not work. People are hurting and want to be heard, not just given a prescription during a five-minute visit. Everyone is unique. Meeting families where they are in their health journey to move them forward is my goal. I was left on this earth after stage 3B breast cancer not to just get well myself, but to use my new insight to help others in preventing disease and restoring their health to whatever extent the body is able.

Are you or a loved one trapped in the box? Did a story resonate with you? I hope that this book provided you with some insight into how to guide your family back to wellness as well as provoked you to continue to ask the hard questions. I hope that this book is used as a guide to help others who are stuck in the box and are trying to break free to a new level of health freedom, but also that some curious health providers may read it and open their mind to other possibilities. The true heroes in the stories I have told are the children and their supportive, sacrificing families who did not give up hope and were dedicated to sometimes difficult treatment plans.

The Cycle of Illness and the 7Rs of Healing tool is a great place to start, providing a framework for addressing chronic health issues. I've found it to be a reliable way to structure a person's health narrative and share my insights on some of the toughest health challenges I encounter.

Finding an integrative medicine practitioner to help you on your family's health journey is the next step! Never stop questioning. Never stop being a true advocate for your child's health. They are our future, and we cannot fail them!

In Love and Health,

Deborah Z. Bain, MD

References

Abrams, S. A., Albin, J. L., & Landrigan, P. J. (2024). Use of genetically modified organism (GMO)-containing food products in children. *Pediatrics*, *153*(1). https://doi.org/10.1542/ peds.2023-064774

American Psychiatric Association. (2022). *Diagnostic and statistical manual of mental disorders* (5th ed., text rev.). https://doi.org/10.1176/appi.books. 9780890425787

Bernardo, J. F. & Edwards, M. R. (2023) Aluminum toxicity. *Medscape*. https://emedicine. medscape.com/article/165315-overview?form=fpf

Centers for Disease Control and Prevention (2024). Data and statistics on tourette syndrome. https://www.cdc.gov/tourette-syndrome/data/index.html

Daley, M. F., Reifler, L. M., Glanz, J. M., Hambidge, S. J., Getahun, D., Irving, S. A., Nordin, J. D., McClure, D. L., Klein, N. P., Jackson, M. L., Kamidani, S., Duffy, J., & DeStefano, F. (2023). Association between aluminum exposure from vaccines before age 24 months and persistent asthma at age 24 to 59 months. *Academic Pediatrics*, *23*(1), 37-46. https://doi.org/10.1016/j.acap.2022.08.006

Davidson, K. P. (2022). The Association of Nocturnal Enuresis and Breathing Disorders in Children with Sleep Disordered Breathing: A retrospective review of pediatric cases treated with a preformed monoblock oral appliance. *Journal of Sleep Disorders & Therapy*, *11*(1).

Demarque, D., Jouanny, J., Poitevin, B., & Saint-Jean, Y. (2007). *Pharmacology and homeopathic materia medica*. CEDH International.

Doherty, T. S., & Carroll, A. E. (2020). Believing in overcoming cognitive biases. *AMA Journal of Ethics*, *22*(9), 773-778. https://doi.org/10.1001/amajethics.2020.773

Drugs.com. https://www.drugs.com/

Dumais, J.-M. (2023). Baby who died 34 hours after vaccines had toxic level of aluminum in his blood, report confirms. *The Defender*. https://childrenshealthdefense.org/defender/maine- baby-sawyer-vaccine-death-aluminum/

Gianoni-Capenakas, S., Gomes, A. C., Mayoral, P., Miguez, M., Pliska, B., & Lagravere, M. (2020). Sleep-disordered breathing: The dentists' role: A systematic review. *Journal of Dental Sleep Medicine*, *7*(1). http://dx.doi.org/10.15331/jdsm.7108

Golden, I. (2010). *Vaccination & homeoprophylaxis?: A review of risks and alternatives* (7th ed.). Isaac Golden Publications.

Grippaudo, C., Paolantonio, E. G., Antonini, G., Saulle, R., La Torre, G., & Deli, R. (2016). Association between oral habits, mouth breathing, and malocclusion. *Acta Otorhinolaryngologica Italica*, *36*(5), 386-394. https://doi.org/10.14639/0392-100X-770

Hooker, B. S., & Miller, N. Z. (2020). Analysis of health outcomes in vaccinated and unvaccinated children: Developmental delays, asthma, ear infections and gastrointestinal disorders. *SAGE Open Medicine*, *8*. https://doi.org/10.1177/2050312120925344

Houlihan, J., Kropp, T., Wiles, R., Gray, S., Campbell, C., & Greene, A. (2005). Body burden: The pollution in newborns. *Environmental Working Group.* https://www.ewg.org/ research/body-burden-pollution-newborns

Jaiswal, Y. S., & Williams, L. L. (2017). A glimpse of Ayurveda: The forgotten history and principles of Indian traditional medicine. *Journal of Traditional and Complementary Medicine*, *7*(1), 50-53. https://doi.org/10.1016/j.jtcme.2016.02.002

Kadar, N., Romero, R., & Papp, Z. (2018). Ignaz Semmelweis: The "savior of mothers" on the 200th anniversary of his birth. *American Journal of Obstetrics and Gynecology*, *219*(6), 519-522. https://doi.org/10.1016/j.ajog.2018.10.036

Lipman, Z. M., Labib, A., & Yosipovitch, G. (2021). Current clinical options for the management of itch in atopic dermatitis. *Clinical, Cosmetic and Investigational Dermatology*, *2021*(14), 959-969. https://doi.org/10.2147/CCID.S289716

Lyons-Weiler, J., McFarland, G., & La Joie, E. (2020). Impact of catch-up vaccination on aluminum exposure due to new laws and post social distancing. *Journal of Trace Elements in Medicine and Biology*, *62*. https://doi.org/10.1016/j.jtemb.2020.126649

Maltese, P. E., Michelini, S., Baronio, M., & Bertelli, M. (2019). Molecular foundations of chiropractic therapy. *Acta Biomedica*, *90*(10), 93-102. https://doi.org/10.23750/abm. v90i10-S.8768

Mawson, A. R., Ray, B. D., Bhuiyan, A. R., & Jacob, B. (2016). Vaccination and health outcomes: A survey of 6- to 12-year-old vaccinated and unvaccinated children based on mothers' reports. Initially published in *Frontiers in Public Health*. https://jeffreydachmd.com/wp-content/uploads/2018/08/Health-Outcomes-6-12-year-old-Vaccinated-and-Unvaccinated-based-on-Mothers-Reports-Mawson-AR-Front-Public-Health-2016.pdf

Miller, N. Z. (2016). Combining childhood vaccines at one visit is not safe. *Journal of American Physicians and Surgeons*, *21*(2), 47-49. https://www.researchgate.net/publication/304896973_Combining_Childhood_Vaccines_at_One_Visit_Is_Not_Safe

Miller, N. Z. (2021). Vaccines and sudden infant death: An analysis of the VAERS database 1990–2019 and review of the medical literature. *Toxicology Reports*, *8*, 1324-1335. https://doi.org/10.1016/j.toxrep.2021.06.020

National Center for Environmental Health (2023). Asthma: Most recent national asthma data. *Centers for Disease Control and Prevention*. https://www.cdc.gov/asthma/most_recent_national_asthma_data.htm

National Center for Immunization and Respiratory Diseases (2023). Vaccine recommendations and guidelines of the ACIP: Contraindications and precautions. *Centers for Disease Control and Prevention*. https://www.cdc.gov/vaccines/hcp/acip-recs/general-recs/contraindications.html

Orient, J. M. (1999). Mandating vaccines: Government practicing medicine without a license? *Medical Sentinel*, 4(5), 166-168. https://www.vaccineinfo.net/issues/vaccinemandates/nomandates.shtml

Price, W. A. (2009). *Nutrition and physical degeneration*. Price Pottenger Nutrition. (Original work published 1939).

Rakel, D. (2018). *Integrative medicine* (4th ed.). Elsevier.

Seneff, S. (2021). *Toxic legacy: How the weedkiller glyphosate is destroying our health and the environment*. Chelsea Green Publishing Company.

Samsel, A., & Seneff, S. (2016). Glyphosate pathways to modern diseases V: Amino acid analogue of glycine in diverse proteins. *Journal of Biological Physics and Chemistry*, *16*(1), 9-46. https://doi.org/10.4024/03SA16A.jbpc.16.01

Shaw, W. (2013). Evidence that increased acetaminophen use in vulnerable children appears to be a major cause of the epidemics of autism, attention deficit with hyperactivity, and asthma. *Journal of Restorative Medicine*, *2*(1), 14-29. https://doi.org/10.14200/jrm.2013.2.0101

Snider, P. & Zeff, J. (2019). Unifying principles of naturopathic medicine *origins and definitions*. *Integrative Medicine*, *18*(4), 36-39. ncbi.nlm.nih.gov/pmc/articles/PMC7219457/

Vasquez, A., Baker, S. M., Bennett, P., Bland, J. S., Galland, L., Hedaya, R. J., Houston, M., Hyman, M., Lombard, J., & Rountree, R. (2010). *Textbook of functional medicine 2010*. Example Product Manufacturer.

Watad, A., David, P., Brown, S., & Shoenfeld, Y. (2017). Autoimmune/inflammatory syndrome induced by adjuvants and thyroid autoimmunity. *Frontiers in Endocrinology*, *7*(150), 1-5. https://doi.org/10.3389/fendo.2016.00150

Zablotsky, B., Black, L. I., & Akinbami, L. J. (2023). Diagnosed allergic conditions in children aged 0-17 years: United States, 2021. *National Center for Health Statistics*, 459. https://www.cdc.gov/nchs/data/databriefs/db459.pdf

Notes

Notes

Notes

Notes

Notes

Made in the USA
Monee, IL
04 November 2026

67383621R00075